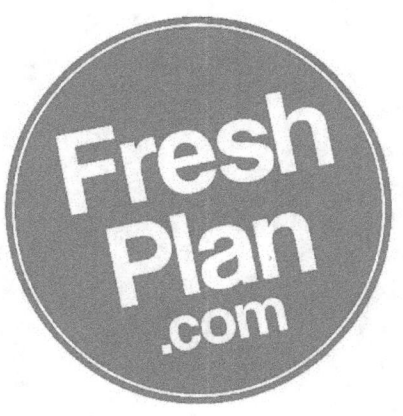

The Freshplan Diet by Carl Harris

STOP FAILING AND START LOSING WEIGHT!

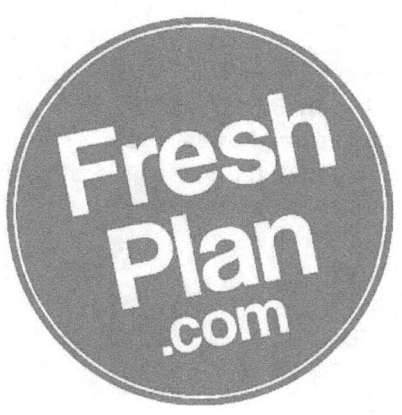

Change Your Life Forever!
Join the Freshplan Revolution Today

By Carl Harris

Published in 2015 by X22 Ltd

Copyright © 2015 by Carl Harris

First published 2015

ISBN-13: 978-1519205490

ISBN-10: 151920549X

Published By X22 Limited Trading as X22 Books
www.x22books.co.uk

For my wonderful family who gave me the inspiration to change my life. My loving partner Sharon for putting up with me for 20 years, without you I am nothing.

The Freshplan Diet by Carl Harris

"No one is truly happy being fat, the best you can achieve is to be happy despite being fat. The path to true happiness is to learn how to lose weight and the skills to manage your weight for life."

Carl Harris

The Freshplan Diet by Carl Harris

Introduction

HI, I'M CARL HARRIS. I USED TO BE FAT, UNFIT AND REALLY UNHEALTHY!

I had just turned 42, and I was laying in my hospital bed, having just been told for the second time in three years I had suffered a Pulmonary Embolism (PE), a potentially fatal blood clot on the lung. Tears rolled down my face at the thought that, unless I sorted myself out, I would not be around to see my daughter grow up.

I weighed in excess of 20 stone (280 pounds), I constantly felt dreadful, physically and mentally, and I couldn't remember the last time I was able to look in the mirror, or indeed, what it felt like to feel fit and healthy. That was my rock bottom but I made a decision that night, one that not only changed my life, but gave me back my life.

The decision I made was a simple one, to make some big changes. I regard myself as intelligent (I hold an honours degree), I have achieved a lot in my life to date, both in business and personally, and have read more self-help books than most. The self-pity I felt at the start of the night had turned to self-anger by the morning. *How the hell had I let myself get into this state?* As the old saying goes, I had 'let myself go a bit'.

The truth of the matter, which I didn't realise back then, is I never actually had control of myself to begin with, and I have been fighting a losing battle, as most overweight people have, with food and weight all of my life. I could visualise the person I wanted to be; slim, fit and healthy. At that moment, that person was nothing more than a distant dream.

I realised I needed to make a change, there and then. Although I am not a fan of his, the lyrics from the Michael Jackson song, 'Man in the Mirror', kept playing themselves in my head:

> *'I'm Gonna Make A Change,*
> *For Once In My Life*
> *It's Gonna Feel Real Good,*
> *Gonna Make A Difference*
> *Gonna Make It Right . . .'*
> *Michael Jackson, Man in the Mirror, 1988*

I quickly stopped feeling sorry for myself and decided to grab the second (well third, and in all probability, my final) chance in life and **'MAKE THAT CHANGE'**. I decided right then and there that the person I wanted to be was the person I was going to be. It really was, for me, a case of 'Do or Die'. That night, I set some personal objectives, which I emailed to myself from my iPhone:

1. **Lose weight NOW you FAT BASTARD!**
2. **Sort your head out and FAST, FFS!**
3. **Work out why are you are so F***ing FAT and UNHEALTHY!**
4. **Two PE's??? One is just unlucky; two isn't. WTF caused it!**
5. **Dissect every aspect of your life and put it back together so it works properly!**
6. **Live Long and Prosper!**

I had hit rock bottom. No question. Writing those six points in York District Hospital was probably the best thing I have ever done for myself. It started a journey, one of amazing discovery, enlightenment and achievement. A journey from rock bottom to experiencing highs I never thought I would.

Three years later, I am now fit, well, healthy and happy, and four stone (and counting) lighter. I have developed the Freshplan, and it will help you lose weight, keep it off, and live a much healthier and happier life. I promise that you will have a better relationship with food than you have ever had.

I found out what caused me to have two potentially fatal blood clots. There is no doubt in my mind that it was my addiction, (I can now call it that) to Diet Cola. I would drink several cans a day, thinking it had no calories and was perfectly safe. I was wrong!

Research has found that people who drink diet soft drinks daily are 43 percent more likely to suffer a vascular event, including a stroke. As a heavy user, this risk is even greater. I can now say I was addicted to it, and it almost killed me. I genuinely thought addiction issues related to tobacco, alcohol and drugs; you know, stuff that can actually kill you! But the reality is we, as a culture, are addicted to the food we eat, as well as what we drink. These drinks that are supposed to be good for you are actually not at all. The so-called diet or 'lite' versions are actually more harmful for you, and certainly just as, if not more, addictive than the fully loaded versions.

The reason we are getting fatter is because the manufactured and convenience food we eat is really bad for us and it is designed to get us hooked on eating more of it. We crave it. Our desire to eat it is stronger than our desire to not have it and lose weight. That part of our brain that drives craving and addiction is five times more powerful than the part of our brain that wants to lose weight and be healthy.

The food manufacturers are designing food to stimulate our brain's pleasure receptors. Our desire to consume it wins every time and there, in a nutshell, is the cause of the worldwide obesity epidemic. The perfect storm. Cheap and widely available food, full of stuff that makes us fat and unhealthy, which we are addicted to eating!

I felt like a big fat failure for years. I desperately wanted to lose weight, but I just seemed to fail constantly. I could never stick to it. I have been a slave to my cravings and zero willpower for years. I tried every diet, all the latest fads; you name it, I have tried it. I have lost weight, but ultimately, put it back on. I have never had the willpower to say NO when the cravings came calling. If this sounds familiar, let me lift a huge burden from your mind. You are not a failure. You never had much of a chance, and there is more good news. We can win the war. We have the power!

You are in possession of the most powerful weight loss weapon in the world, your mind. Right now, it is working against you because most of us do not know how to use it to achieve our objective of losing weight.

The Freshplan will unlock limitless potential and liberate you from the burden of being overweight, unhappy and unhealthy and from the persistent self-sabotage of our attempts to lose weight. The big secret is it is actually really easy when you know how!

It sounds daunting and complicated, doesn't it? But it is not. I will show you how, once you take back control, there will be no stopping you, and your life will change forever. You will embark on a journey where the destination is a thinner, healthier and happier you with a brighter outlook on life. All I can tell you is that where I am now, compared to where I was when I was lying in that hospital bed just over three years ago, is beyond anything I could ever have wished for.

I have made the journey from despair to happiness, and now, it's your turn to banish the old you and build the new and improved you with the Freshplan. It is a cliché to say you only get one life, but it is true. However, you have a second chance to live what is left of it, on your own terms, as the person you desire to be. Change happens only by design, but when you make key changes to your diet, your weight and your health, then the direction of your life will consequentially change for the better.

If you make a commitment to yourself today to lose weight forever, you will do it with the Freshplan. Failing will be a thing of the past. It will not be hard, painful, complicated, time consuming or expensive (except maybe buying new, smaller clothes).

It will, however, be enjoyable, enlightening, liberating and very easy! If I can do it, then anyone can, believe me! Let me show you just how easy it really is to lose weight and keep it off for good.

Carl J Harris BA HONS, DDM

Change Your Life Forever!
Join the Freshplan Revolution

The Freshplan mindset

The Freshplan PELOS diet

Chapter 1
No one really likes being fat

Chances are, if you are reading this book, then you want to lose weight or live a healthier life. Human nature is such that I can confidently say, if you are fat, (overweight or obese), you will not be happy about it, and being unhappy due to weight issues has negative effects on other aspects of your life. You want to make a change.

The human brain is simply not designed to be happy in a fat body. I hear people say they are fat, but they are happy. Who are they kidding? Probably no one other than themselves. Fat Shaming is a contemporary term, but in my experience, as a former fat person, no one can ever shame you more than you are ashamed of yourself.

Plus size fashion is now big business, which I find very sad. It is an acceptance that the battle against obesity is lost. You can call it whatever you want, plus size, outsize, over size, big and tall, but there is no getting away from it. If it looks like a fat person, it is a fat person. Give anyone a choice, and they will choose thin over fat every time. There is a thin person inside everyone, waiting to get out.

If you disagree or are offended by that statement, and you are GENUINELY happy being fat (overweight, big, cuddly, curvy or plus size, call it what you will), and do not want to change, then this book is not for you! I am not here to judge anyone. I am here to help people who want to make a change. The choice is yours to make, and if you are fat by choice, and it makes you happy, then that is your choice to make. I ask you just one thing. Please let me know if you are, because I have never met anyone who is GENUINELY (and not just saying it) happy being fat!

Saying you are happy being fat is just another excuse for repeatedly failing at dieting. No one ever sets out to be fat, but usually people who keep failing at losing weight simply accept defeat. Saying they are happy being fat really means they have come to terms with their inability to become the thin person they desire to be. Even with a rudimentary understanding of human psychology, you can confidently say that fat and happy are complete contradictions.

The statistics surrounding weight in the UK are eye watering. According to research firm Mintel, in 2013 there were 29 million UK adults who tried to lose weight. Official statistics show 61 percent of the UK population are still overweight, and staggeringly, more than 15 million (in 2014) are classed clinically obese. As a nation, we are eating ourselves to death. The statistics for the UK alone are unbelievable...

- 61% of the UK population are overweight (including kids)
- 25% are obese
- 29m people try to lose weight every year
- 65% of all women and 44% of all men want to lose weight
- Only 5% of women say they are not conscious of their weight
- Only 17% of men say they are not conscious of their weight

- £2bn is spent on diet food products in the UK every year
- 85% of dieters fail and get fatter.

These figures are growing at an alarming rate. Already, we can say the majority of people in the UK are overweight, and a quarter of the population is obese. The Independent newspaper reported recently that by 2030, there will be 26 million people in the UK who are obese - a rise of 73% in only 15 years. It is a huge problem. The government is trying to educate us; the Five a Day Campaign has raised awareness but their advertising budget of a few million pounds is dwarfed by the billions the food companies spend, and the healthy message just gets drowned out.

It is a losing battle, not just in the UK, but on a global scale. Almost every developed economy has a weight problem, ranging in size. The statistics for the USA dwarf those of the UK. Not surprising when you can buy cola in half gallon cups. If you have never seen Supersize Me, a film by Morgan Spurlock, I urge you to watch it.

We live in a social paradox where media advertising has created the aspiration to be young, slim, and have a beautiful body, yet the trend is going in the completely opposite direction at an alarming rate. Something is going badly wrong.

Diets, diet clubs, and diet books are making big money, yet they are badly failing their customers, because only a minority ever succeed. Losing weight is something people are finding almost impossible to achieve. They set out with good intentions but it is not long before they self-sabotage those efforts, and usually, end up putting on weight.

The problem is what we eat. Modern day society has a diet based on supermarket food, produced in high volume with the constant pressure of keeping the price down. Most of the food the average person eats is manufactured or processed (by that I mean, not fresh natural food), and that is the root cause of why we get fat, stay fat and despite longing to take positive action to lose weight, we are constantly failing. Why do we fail when it comes to dieting? The answer is simple. We are not in control of our ability to resist eating processed food. We are addicted at differing levels but unless we break the cycle of addiction, we will never lose weight.

If you have failed over and over again with diets and losing weight, clearly you need to adopt a fundamentally fresh approach. It was Einstein who said doing the same thing over and over, expecting different results, is the definition of insanity.

SO WHY IS LOSING WEIGHT SO HARD?

Actually it is not; it is really easy! There is no secret to it. Take in fewer calories than you burn on a daily basis, job done. Just about everyone who wants to lose weight is 'starting tomorrow,' but tomorrow never comes. Tomorrow just brings more of the same and an expanding waist line.

Dieters set out with good intentions but almost always fail. The diet industry is worth millions, but has an 85% failure rate. Just pause a moment to take that in. 85% of people who start a diet, fail.

Not only do 85% of people who embark on a diet fail, they actually weigh more than when they started after only three months. The civilised world is getting fatter; the term 'OBESITY EPIDEMIC' is now commonly used and is no longer disputed. Humans put on weight easily but seem unable to lose it and maintain a healthy weight. As the world gets fatter, the more the diet industry rakes in. Can you think of another industry that is thriving on the back of failing 85% of its customers?

People become so desperate to lose weight they resort to extreme and dangerous measures in ever increasing numbers. The NHS performs around 8,000 'bariatric' procedures each year.

Gastric band surgery, effectively removing a large portion of the stomach, is growing at a rapid rate, but is a pretty brutal and last resort form of weight reversal. In 2014, a 12 year old girl had this surgery on the NHS. Such is our inability to lose weight, desperate people take desperate measures.

In 2015, six British people died after taking diet pills containing highly toxic chemicals, which they bought over the internet. It is so sad to read these type of reports that are becoming all too frequent. How has it come to this?

I cannot save the world, but I can help you save yourself and opt out of obesity with the Freshplan.

I am going to guess you have been on a diet before. You either were unable to stick to it long enough to lose weight, or you lost weight but soon put it back on. I am no Mystic Meg. That is a statement that applies to almost everyone who is overweight.

The odds are stacked against you, before you ever even start a diet. A lethal combination of the food you eat, the way your mind works, and the lifestyle you lead all conspire to make failure inevitable. It becomes a vicious circle of diet, fail, eat more, and get fatter, until we set out again, expecting different results that never materialise. Then eventually, you accept defeat and give up.

The craving for processed food is too strong for most people to resist, but it is designed to get you hooked. Although you want to say no, you end up giving in, because you have a voice in your brain that drives you to want it so badly. The part of your brain that drives this is five times more powerful than the part of you that wants to lead a healthy, thinner life. You probably put this down to having no willpower but your mind is in constant conflict, and as far as your weight is concerned, it is working against you and doing you more harm than good. Not anymore. The Freshplan will teach you how to break the cycle and put you in total control of your weight for life!

The Freshplan is designed to show you how adopting the right mindset will give you the willpower to succeed. You will create a new and improved, self-disciplined version of yourself, who has the power to easily lose weight and keep it off for life. You can break out of that vicious cycle of failure and despair and become the person you always wanted to be.

Unless you change your mindset, you will keep failing. I quickly realised everything I thought I knew about food and nutrition was wrong. You will be amazed how simple losing weight actually is when you get willpower on your side. It is no wonder we are getting fat when we have no idea what we are eating and what we should be eating. Everyone starts a diet with good intentions but good intentions need to be supported with positive actions. Most people give up at the first sign of 'failure'. The truth is, no one actually wants to go on a diet, but they know they need to. Because of how your mind is currently wired to work, you find it almost impossible to stick to it because you have failed before you start, with completely the wrong mindset, which in itself guarantees only one outcome; FAILURE.

"I have failed over and over again in life. That is why I succeed."
Michael Jordan

It is more than a vicious circle. It is a downward spiral that can lead to low self-esteem and depression. I can understand why people reach the stage where they will try anything! Over the years, I have tried probably every diet going and always failed. Like most people, I blamed the diet for my failure, rather than my inability to follow it and make it work for me. Have you ever heard anyone actually say something along the lines of:
"A lot of people have lost weight following this diet, but I was not resolute or strong enough to follow simple instructions, and I am in fact, now fatter than when I started. I found it easier to blame the diet than accept personal responsibility for my failure."

Neither have I but that is the reality. I have heard plenty of *excuses* as to why people are fat and don't do anything about it. Hey, I have probably used them all myself at one time or another. **The first thing you need to give up to lose weight are the excuses.** Once you have the Freshplan mindset there are no excuses that will hold water. Whatever excuse(s) you are hiding behind for not being able to lose weight, I will wager that even you don't really believe them. I say to people; you have to make a choice:

"To become thin and healthy, you either stop making excuses and get on with it, or you live with excuses and keep getting fatter!"

Sometimes, tough love is the kindest approach. You want to lose weight but can't. With the Freshplan, you will change that for good. Losing weight is actually a simple process and boils down to only four words, *"EAT LESS, MOVE MORE"*. It sounds so easy, doesn't it?

With the Freshplan mindset that is as simple as it needs to be. Think of a diet as an investment in yourself, your loved ones and the people that love you. You will feel better, and that will make you a better person to be around. You will also be more energetic and live longer and when you lose weight and keep it off, you will become a figure of inspiration. Even the people you know, who were secretly wanting you to fail, because they can't do it, will even concede that you have done well. The Freshplan will be life changing, which is in no way underestimating the impact that losing weight and being healthy will have.

You don't need me to tell you that saying it is one thing, doing it another altogether. You will, no doubt, be sceptical. Fair enough, but what is the worst that can happen? You try it, fail again, and are no worse off than when you started! But that is not going to happen. The Freshplan tackles the real reason you fail at losing weight, your lack of willpower and self-discipline. The Freshplan is more than just another diet; it's a Mindset and a lifestyle plan that gets you thin and healthy and keeps you that way for life.

I felt like a failure for years. But let me share with you one key fact. **You are not a failure!** The odds are so stacked against you, because of what is in our food, when you start a diet, you cannot be blamed for failing. Simply choosing to go on a diet or joining a diet club is not enough. Before you ever start the physical process of losing weight, you need to address the root cause of past failures, understand why you got fat, why you have been unable to lose the weight, and of course, what to do about it.

Chapter 2
You are hard-wired to fail at diets

Most dieters fail, not because they do not want to lose weight. Everyone aspires to be thin, fit and healthy. We fail badly at dieting, not because we are weak or stupid. It is because our brain is working against us. Once you understand the processes your mind goes through in relation to food, desire and habits, then you have a starting point.

Willpower failure is the reason we can't stick to a diet plan. This was always my problem. I could always hear a voice in my head, sabotaging my good intentions. I always felt conflicted when I had a craving for food, almost like I had a devil in my head urging me to 'have it, go on. You know you want it'. I never understood why I would always give in so easily.

Then I read a book in 2012 called *The Chimp Paradox* by Dr Steve Peters (Random House), which was a turning point for me. The premise of the book is if you manage your mind in the right way, you become unstoppable, and anything you want to achieve is possible. The obstacle preventing you from reaching your goals is the very thing that ensures you can not only achieve them, but surpass them. The Freshplan shows you how to manage your mind, change your habits and take control of all aspects of food and weight management. A few simple changes will have an unbelievable impact on your life!

Your brain is hugely complex, sophisticated and powerful. It is the most powerful computer on Earth. Just like a computer, you have an operating system. In technology, this is called software or firmware, to be more specific.

"In electronic systems and computing, firmware is a tangible electronic component with embedded software instructions. Typically, they are used to tell an electronic device how to operate. Most firmware can now be updated."
Wikipedia definition.

Although it is much more complicated in the brain, essentially, we all have our own unique firmware, or mindware, which dictates how we operate. Your brain's mindware is constantly updating itself without you noticing (subconsciously). This is the key to understanding your entire relationship with food and what goes on in your mind, preventing you from losing weight and keeping it off. The great news is, though, that your mindware can be easily reprogrammed, by you, to create a new and improved version (Me Version 2), who will achieve your weight loss objectives. You know what they say:

"When you put your [improved] mind to it, anything is possible!"

I made a commitment to myself to lose weight and to make sure it never came back. Over the last three years, I have done extensive research to develop, analyse and modify the Freshplan. I have, personally, put everything I am advising into practice and it works. A series of small changes that add up to a big difference in your life is the foundation which underpins the Freshplan.

If this sounds familiar, I got the idea from Sir Dave Brailsford, who transformed British Cycling from nothing into an unstoppable force of world domination. He believed in a concept that he referred to as the:

"Aggregation of marginal gains."
Sir Dave Brailsford

He explained it as, "The one percent margin for improvement in everything you do." His belief was if you improved every area related to cycling by just 1 percent, then those small gains would add up to remarkable improvement. He was proved right. The Freshplan applies the same logic to weight loss, providing you with a blueprint, taking you through a series of easy steps to achieve your objectives of losing weight and personal goals, which you can maintain for life.

The Freshplan will put you in control, often for the first time in your life, giving you the POWER to decide what to eat and always be the weight you want to be.

I'M JUST AN ORDINARY BLOKE, BUT I'VE GOT THE T-SHIRT...

I would like to make it clear that I am not a doctor, dietician, psychologist, psychiatrist, pharmacist, sociologist, nutritionist, chemist, biologist, scientist or anything that ends in -ist. I have probably tried every diet going over the last 25 years, and suffered all the problems overweight people face. I have learned the hard way and discovered what it takes to overcome obesity. I have tried every which way to lose weight in the past and have produced a plan that works.

My struggle with food and weight could have cost me my life, which is no exaggeration. One day, I hit rock bottom and then turned my life around. It has not been easy. I have had setbacks along the road but from what I have achieved, I have created a blueprint for you to follow. I have not only thoroughly studied and researched all aspects of diet and weight management to create the Freshplan, but I have also successfully practiced it, losing and maintaining weight loss in excess of four stone. Every day used to be a battle with food; now it isn't. The Freshplan is the most liberating experience which will lift a huge burden from your life. It is time for you to banish being overweight forever and rediscover happiness.

The dark cloud of gloom and failure, which hangs over you, is about to clear. A ray of light will shine upon you. We all feel better when the sun is shining!

So I may not have formal qualifications but I have been there, seen it, done it, and got the t-shirt. I was told by a newly qualified doctor that he studied nutrition for no more than two days during his six years of training. I found an article about twin Doctors, Alexander and Chris Van Tulleken, who gave up fat and sugar for a month for a BBC programme. They are quoted in the Daily Mail:

"But here's the problem: despite being doctors - I also have a degree in public health - neither of us knew much about losing weight and eating healthily. These topics fall between the cracks at medical school. Yes, we understood biochemistry and food metabolism and knew a lot about the consequences of being overweight. But which diets work, why we eat too much, and why losing weight is so hard don't sit within any medical speciality."

Amazing, given obesity is the biggest risk factor facing the nation's health. GP's are on the frontline, and there is no question the biggest driver of fatal disease is easily obesity.

I have waded through the mountain of complex and conflicting nutrition and diet advice to produce an easy plan to lose weight and stay thin for life. I have studied how the mind works and why it is the single, biggest barrier to weight loss. I have done the hard yards, had successes, failures, setbacks and have come out the other side. Believe me, if I can lose weight, get healthy and stay that way, then so can you!

Chapter 3
What is the Freshplan?

The Freshplan is an integrated life management plan, which can be applied to many aspects of your life and business. With Freshplan, you can unlock your full potential because the only person holding you back is you. The Freshplan gives you a more positive and effective Mindset, coupled with smarter practical application, providing you with a strategic, integrated end-to-end solution with quantifiable results. The Freshplan was developed, initially, for weight loss and weight management, but is now being applied as an easy to use turnkey solution to achieve a wide spectrum of personal and business objectives.

This is the Freshplan Weight Management Plan. The Freshplan Mindset makes achieving your goals and objectives possible by restructuring your approach to weight loss. Clearly, if willpower has not worked, then without fundamentally changing your approach, you will not transform from a failure to a loser, a weight loser! Once you have the right mindset in place, the Freshplan gives you a smart and effective way to reach your personal objectives and goals.

Your objectives are quantifiable and measurable. Your goals are personal to you. They are your personal reasons and motivations. Once you have specified these goals, the Freshplan will get you there through a structured, strategic and smart approach, specifically aimed to illuminate failure and get you to a successful outcome as quickly and painlessly as possible. The philosophy that underpins The Freshplan is to work smarter not harder. By being smarter, you don't need to work as hard, and you can reach your personal goals, which are of course, both realistic and achievable.

The Freshplan Weight Loss and Management Solution is an integrated approach, combining mindset and diet. This is not just another diet; clearly, just being on a diet has not been enough to lose weight in the past. Freshplan is not a fad or an extreme weight loss craze. The Freshplan is a long-term plan for you to change, for life. Yo-yo dieting is a thing of the past. The Freshplan gives you a complete toolkit to enable you to make that lifestyle change and be in control of the food you eat and your weight, rather than the other way round. You will upgrade yourself to the new improved, fit, healthy and happy person you have always wanted to be.

I have written this book in two parts.

1 The Freshplan Mindset and Weight Loss Toolkit

The Freshplan Mindset gives back the control over what, where, when and why you eat. You will be armed with the willpower, as well as a highly effective toolkit of tips, tricks and information to be a success and lose weight. You will learn how to reverse years of willpower failure, finally being able to stick to a diet. You will no longer sabotage your own efforts to lose weight.

You will learn why you have failed for years at losing weight and why the food you eat is doing more than just making you fat. The Freshplan will completely change your mindset in both your conscious and subconscious mind, making weight loss and weight management an almost automatic process. You will no longer be conflicted between your desire to lose weight and the more powerful food cravings that have always put paid to any hope of achieving it.

The diet clubs and books tell you what to eat and when. They tell you to use willpower and positive thinking to see it through. Willpower has been something easier said than done, until now! Without the Freshplan mindset, you will remain in the same vicious cycle where diets make you hungry; you crave more of the processed food, chemically optimised for maximum desire, and it is inevitably only a matter of time before you give in and end up eating more of it than you did before.

It is logical that if you are overweight, frustrated, and unable to successfully lose weight, no matter how hard you try and how many times you repeat the process, there is a problem somewhere. There is no magic switch that changes everything instantly, just because you decide to go on a diet. If you have ever felt like you are possessed by something inside your head that makes you eat and sabotage your diet, then you are right!

If you have failed at dieting, even once, without changing your mindset, you are almost guaranteed to fail again and again. Even if you lose weight, you are highly likely to put it back on, unless you understand and can control your food mindset.

"The Freshplan Mindset transforms your 85% chance of failure into an 85% chance of success."

Simply by reprogramming your mind's firmware (mindware) in very simple ways, you will have a Fresh Mindset, where you understand the processes going on in your mind. The Freshplan has a series of easy to use techniques that will give you the willpower to say NO when you need to say NO.

For most people, the diet journey starts with good intentions, but ends in despair. The story, sadly, all too common is as follows:

- **Good intentions**
- **Followed by self-sabotage (or lack of willpower)**
- **Which leads to self-loathing (feelings of regret and guilt at not sticking to your diet)**
- **Causing great personal frustration and inner conflict (feelings of failure)**
- **Resulting is despair (this is where people often turn to desperate measures)**
- **Start again or...**
- **And ultimately end in failure. (This is when people give up, accept defeat, stay fat or get fatter, and excuse that by claiming they are actually happy).**

I'm going to wager this sounds all too familiar. I spent years trapped in this cycle of despair and failure. However, the good news is the person you want to be, the one who says no to food cravings and is a success at weight loss, is within everyone, including you!

With The Freshplan Mindset, you will start to manage your mind to work effectively towards losing weight and achieving the objectives you set for yourself. You will be in total control, and no matter what diet you then follow, you will achieve results you never thought were possible. Failure will be a thing of the past. It is the most valuable thing you will learn in relation to losing weight.

The Freshplan arms you with the POWER technique to make the right decision and overcome food cravings. The Freshplan Mindset takes you on a journey consisting of three elements:

- **Where are you now?**
- **Where do you want to get?**
- **How are you going to get there?**

First, you have to understand why you have repeatedly been unsuccessful at losing weight. You will gain an understanding of the basics of nutrition and why modern processed foods are designed to be addictive.

You will set your objectives and goals. It is important you know where you want to get to on your journey and what you want to achieve. Once realistic and achievable goals and objectives have been set, you will then embark on your journey.

The Freshplan is structured around a successful formula of objective strategy and tactics, or OST. The strategy is the diet plan you pursue to lose weight. You do not have to use the Freshplan Diet but I would argue it is the simplest and most effective diet you can follow to lose and maintain weight. The Freshplan tactics will teach you how a few small keystone changes will make beneficial changes in your life and achieving your goals. You will learn how to manage weight and your health for life.

There is so much misinformation and ignorance surrounding nutrition that it is important to get an understanding of the food you eat and why modern manufactured food does more harm than good.

Modern processed food has us all hooked. It is designed to hit the bliss point in your brain. The goblin is wide awake in our heads and is much more powerful when it comes to food than we are. We can't kill the goblin, but we can put him back in the box pretty quickly and take control.

It may sound like the Freshplan will give you a totally new personality. You will still be you. People will notice no difference at all, only the size of your waistline and your positive outlook on life. There is no hypnosis (does that even actually work?) involved or any other new age techniques. Knowledge is power and the Freshplan gives you the knowledge and power to succeed.

The Freshplan is so easy you will wonder why you didn't do it years ago. But it is never too late to be the person you always wanted to be. You can then choose to apply the Freshplan Mindset to another diet or follow what I believe is the easiest, most effective, healthy and sensible diet known to man, The Freshplan Diet.

The Freshplan Diet and Weight Management Plan

Once you have adopted the Freshplan Mindset, you will be ready to start shedding those pounds. There are literally thousands of diet options available on the market, some very good, some not so good, some downright dangerous.

Having done so much work and research and by applying what I have learned, I have devised an easy, healthy and sustainable plan to get you to your desired weight and help you stay there for good. As someone who loves food more than most, I believe, above all, life is for living, and food is one of the greatest pleasures we have. Therefore, I would describe The Freshplan Diet as a food lover's diet. We are all human, and I have never lost site of one key fact:

"Energy powers success and leads to a better life"

I am the weight I want to be, I eat out a lot, and I treat myself to the foods I have always enjoyed from time to time, but always maintain my weight. I have just returned from a family holiday to Dubai, where the food in the hotel was out of this world. I enjoyed a cooked breakfast every day, afternoon tea of scones and cakes, and five star gourmet evening meals. One week after coming home, I am exactly the same weight I was before I left. I am in control and it feels great.

The Freshplan will show you how to lose weight the natural way and how to keep it off for life. The Freshplan Diet is the simplest way to eat and you can choose the foods you love.

This is how the Freshplan works. It's about balance and control. There are two important phases to the Fresh Diet:

1. **Getting to your target weight**
2. **Staying at your target weight for good.**

Phase 1 – The dreaded 'D' word!

Unfortunately, there is no getting away from it. To lose weight, you need to go on a diet. But it will be easy because you will have the Fresh Mindset working for you, and the plan I have devised also tastes great! In fact, rather than being a chore, you will rediscover your love of food. Wonderful natural flavours will reignite your taste buds. The Freshplan Diet is based on the very simple concept of eating food your body was deigned to eat. We call it the PELOS DIET, which stands for PERSONAL ENERGY LEVEL OUTPUT (for) SUCCESS, a concept we will discuss in detail later.

The food we buy in supermarkets have labels and contains stuff most of us have never heard of. Salt, refined sugar and nasty processed fats feature heavily, and some of the chemicals read more like Walter White's (from TV's *Breaking Bad*) shopping list than something we should be eating. You do not need to label a banana, a carrot or fresh fish. These are fresh foods, as natural as can be, no label required, no processing or anything added. You will be surprised because of how much processed crap you have been eating, how good fresh food or real food, to be more accurate, tastes. The good news is you can eat many of these, even during phase one, in unlimited quantities. Eat more and lose weight! I kid you not, it works!

The Fresh Diet tastes great and not only will you lose weight, but you will notice big improvements in your health and wellbeing. I suffered for many years with bad skin and spots on my back but by switching to a mostly fresh food diet, they disappeared. Blood sugar levels, cholesterol, blood pressure and your resting heart rate will all benefit from the Freshplan PELOS Diet. You will also have much more positive energy than you can ever remember having.

Right, so it's all rabbit food then? Wrong! I just looked back at my food diary and I have had cottage pie, spag-bol, steak, curry and fish and chips. A diet where you eat chips and lose weight, I kid you not. You just have to be smarter about how you make them! We will show you how.

I mentioned my food diary above. This is an important tool. You need to write down what you eat daily to keep a record of your intake, as well as keep a journal of your thoughts, successes and failures. The power of writing things down, even if only a couple of lines a day, is enormously beneficial, as we will learn.

There is no set timescale to phase one, because it depends on where you start. Clearly, if you need to lose seven pounds to get to your target weight, it will be much quicker than if you need to lose seven stone. But it makes no difference, however much you have to lose. You will do it and enjoy getting there. Even if you have setbacks, and I can guarantee almost everyone will, you will get to your target weight.

"The Fresh Mindset with the Freshplan PELOS Diet is too powerful to allow you to fail."

Once you are at your target weight, you will experience a type of euphoria that is hard to rival. I have never (sadly) won the Lottery, but I would expect it comes close to describing the joy I am talking about. It is an amazing feeling to look good and feel fantastic, knowing you have achieved your objectives. The positive effects it has on other areas of your life cannot be underestimated. It is hard to think of any reason you would ever want to go back to the fat version of you. The new you is someone you will love; it is the person you aspire to be. That person is in there right now waiting to get out!

Phase 2 – Keeping it off for life

Phase two is where you maintain your weight, adopting your Fresh Mindset, as well as what you have learned about food and your eating habits to make sure you do not revert to your old ways, you know, the fat, unhealthy and unhappy you!

I call phase two, weight management. Having gotten to your target weight, all the hard work is done. You are now fully equipped to stay thin, and it will, by this time, be second nature for you. Of course, life is never plain sailing, and there are plenty of choppy waters to navigate. I suffered a family bereavement; it was a very difficult time for my family. The old me would have been emotionally triggered to eat and pile on the pounds. By applying the Fresh Mindset, this never happened and despite huge disruption and high emotion, my weight remained the same.

Your new desire to stay thin will be far stronger than your craving to binge on unhealthy food. Researchers in the USA on formerly obese people, who they had helped lose weight, found some of them would rather lose a limb or the sight in one eye than ever be obese again. This may sound like nonsense but it is credible research and illustrates the harmful effect that weight can have on your emotional state. As I said previously, find anyone who would GENUINELY rather be fat than thin and healthy. I have never met anyone who would. I have met plenty who say it, but it doesn't take long for the mask to slip and the reality to manifest itself.

I know what it is like to be at both ends of the spectrum; obese, addicted to Diet Coke, serious health issues, and almost at the point of despair. I am now happy with my weight, fit, healthy and extremely happy. I know which I would choose every time!

LET THE JOURNEY START FOR YOU TODAY!

The Freshplan is the total solution to losing weight and long-term weight management. You can overcome the barriers holding you hostage in an overweight body and take control of your weight, your health and your life.

I make you a simple promise. If you read this book and follow the Freshplan, you will feel better than you have felt in a long time, even perhaps better than you have ever felt. One thing I can say, beyond any doubt, is there is no food known to man that tastes better than it feels to be happy and healthy!

Every journey starts with a single step, you have taken that first step by reading the Freshplan.

Chapter 4
Why is everyone getting fat?

Processed food is really bad for you…

If you have got this far, then it is a fair bet you want to and are ready to lose weight. You will be fired up and ready to start The Freshplan. That is great news but before we do anything, it is important to understand at least the basics about the food we eat and why that is the root cause of your weight problems. Do not skip this section. Read it in full. It is important. You will also be amazed by what comes next!

The reason most of us are getting fat is because we are being fed food that is toxic to our wellbeing. I am not a scientist and you do not need to be or go too deep into it to understand the primary reasons it is so easy to get fat and so hard to lose weight. The problem is simple; processed food, which is more about taste than nutrition. Sugar, sugar substitutes, and manmade fats are the baddies. We eat far too much of them and it's no wonder when they are optimised to get us hooked!

Modern cultures have a diet which is almost exclusively processed food-based. Food is cheap, plentiful and tastes better than ever. The problem is it may taste great but it is so bad for us that we are effectively poisoning ourselves. The world is literally eating itself to death!

My aim in creating the Freshplan was to find a solution to make weight loss and keeping it off for life easy. But my first job was to work out what was making me fat and unhealthy so I could avoid it and find out what I should be eating instead. It's common sense really. If it makes you fat, why eat it? If it makes you ill, don't eat it. But if you are anything like me, you have known that all along. So why do we keep eating more and more? It is almost like we are possessed by a sprite goblin to keep on shovelling it in. There must be a better way, right? Something clearly has gone badly wrong with the modern diet.

"The World Is Full of Fools, Who Never Get It Right."
The Lightning Seeds

I am staggered by how little people know about food and nutrition. You may be thinking you do not fall into this category, but there is a big difference between what people think they know and what they actually know. Most people rely on what they read and hear via the media, or what their mate told them once, and sadly end up with a totally confused and ill-informed version of reality.

I said earlier, everything I thought I knew about food turned out to be wrong. If people really knew about food, nutrition and what makes them fat, then we would solve much of the obesity problem overnight. I now believe manufactured food is deliberately designed to get us addicted and that means more to food manufacturers than providing the nourishment that keeps us healthy. Food labelling only confuses the issue, again, deliberately. The term, junk food, is one I now apply to any food, just about, that has a label on it. They only need labels to tell you what kind of crap you are eating. Think that is a stupid thing to say? Let me put forward my case.

People are eating processed foods in such high quantities that it is poisoning their mind and body. Manufactured food is full of crap. This is very strong language and you are thinking this is ridiculous. How can food we buy from the supermarket, produced by some of the biggest companies in the world, be poisoning us? Well, what I have discovered proves to be exactly the case and, for me, explains everything. You might be on the verge of putting this book down now that I have made that statement but stay with me on this. Not only is it worth your time, I guarantee, when you have finished reading, you will start to look at the label on foods much more than you ever did.

So here we go. I set out the case that processed food is, without doubt, the single biggest cause of ill health and obesity. It is also one of the primary causes so many people fail at dieting. When I refer to processed food, I mean all food that has had some sort of human intervention and things added to it. Of course, not all processed food is bad, just most of it!

I recently spoke to a friend, who I had not seen for a long time. He was genuinely pleased to see me looking much lighter and healthy, but said something I hear all too often: *"Nothing I try seems to work for me. I must have fat genes!"*

His tone was one of frustration. I know how he feels. I used to be exactly the same, living the same nightmare and genuinely I too thought I had the 'fat gene'. It is easier to make an excuse, rather than face the truth. I was fat because I ate too much, ate the wrong foods, did little to no exercise and the unhappier I got, the more I ate. I once said the only pleasure left in my life was food. If I couldn't beat it, I thought I may as well enjoy it and the heavier I became. I outgrew my bathroom scales, which only went to 20 stones.

Processed food just tastes so good doesn't it? I agree, I love the taste of it. If you are anything like me, one biscuit was never enough, two became three, and well, you get the picture. Processed food, like takeaway food, is easy, cheap and has the feel good factor. It gives you a lot of pleasure.

What is on the label?

Food labelling is something most people do not read. The rules are not strict enough, and people are often mislead. In fact, the rules are such that consumers are easily mislead or distracted from the harsh reality. My personal view is food labelling and marketing is the biggest deception perpetrated on mankind, ever. There I go again with the hard hitting, extremist statements!

Low fat foods often have big, bold low fat flashes prominently displayed but the high sugar content may be tucked away in the small print on the back somewhere. I look at it like this; foods only need a label to tell you what has been added and done to it. Fresh foods don't need a list of ingredients and chemicals, do they?

The problem is we have no idea what we are eating, but we know we love the taste of it. If something is made to look like it is healthy, then the perception is it is good for us. If it looks like a duck, and quacks like a duck, then surely it is one. That is how food marketing works, by creating an impression.

I wonder how many people actually read the labels on food and how many of those understand what it says. I never bothered, not least because it is written in the smallest possible print. When you manage to see them and read the ingredients, unless you have a degree in biochemistry, you wouldn't know what most of them were anyway. The French for duck is canard. Understanding food labelling is very canard in my view!

Food labels also show how many calories are in the food. A new European regulation on food labelling came into force on 13th December 2014 controlling all the information you see on food labels, from nutrition labelling and the ingredients list, to the size of the writing used. Nutrition labelling is not compulsory until 2016 but any nutrition labels used now must follow the traffic light format in the regulation. The label includes information on energy per 100g and per portion. Energy is given in both kJ (kilojoules) and kcal (kilocalories). This information was always provided on the back of the pack but is now available (or will be) on the front of the pack too.

Traffic light colours are given to indicate whether a product is high (red), medium (amber) or low (green) in fat, saturates, sugars and salt.

The first problem is what 100g looks like or what a portion is. The rules allow them to vary the quantities to make it look like a food is low calorie.

The almond milk brand I use has two versions, sweetened and unsweetened.

The calories for unsweetened are shown per 200g, and in the sweetened, per 100g. It appears there are twice as many calories in the sweetened version, but the reality (simple maths) is there are actually four times as many. Bending the rules? Not at all. It is perfectly legal to do so. Some clever font size variation and there you go, perception and reality at odds with each other.

I will boldly predict the portion size used is often less than is actually consumed as well. But at least we have some sort of guide. Showing the energy value of a product is useful but only if the consumer is aware of what it is saying. Most people are familiar with the term calorie, which is actually an abbreviation of kilocalorie. If you have ever wondered why there are two units of measurement used, kj and kcal, here is the answer.

Both a kilocalorie and a kilojoule are a measure or unit of the energy in food. The best example is to say they are like miles and kilometres. They measure the same thing, just to a different scale. The common measure amongst consumers is calories. In essence, the number of calories you consume is simply a way of describing the amount of energy your body gets from eating and drinking. Kcals, or kilocalories, are normally referred to simply as calories.

Just to complicate the matter further, however, 1kcal is actually 1,000 calories. So when people refer to something containing 100 calories, it actually has 100,000 calories. It is widely accepted that when calories are quoted, they are, in fact, kilocalories but referred to as calories. Clear as mud, isn't it! Kilojoules or KJS are used mostly by the scientific community. One kcal is equivalent to 4.2 kilojoules. We can disregard those; they are not relevant.

The UK's Department of Health suggests a daily calorie intake of approximately 2,000 calories per day for women and 2,500 for men. It all sounds so simple, doesn't it. I recently was in a shopping centre and my daughter bought a mini portion of fish and chips. The advertising board said only 400 calories per portion, wow, a dieter's dream! I had a fresh salad with mango and crayfish, all fresh ingredients, but with more calories (including the dressing). Which is the better option; fish and chips or a fresh salad? Taking calories here in isolation is completely misleading.

The reason the fish and chips would be a poor weight loss option is they have a high Glycaemic Index (GI). This is a ranking of carbohydrate-containing foods, based on the overall effect on blood glucose levels. Slowly absorbed foods have a low GI rating, while foods that are more quickly absorbed have a higher rating. Carbohydrate foods that are broken down quickly by your body and cause a rapid increase in blood glucose have a high GI rating.

Food broken down quickly by the body means there is excess energy unused by the body, which it stores away as fat. Though measuring fewer calories, the salad was the much better option for the waistline, not to mention being much better nutritionally. You may have heard of the GI Diet. The idea is to eat food with a low GI value. I tried that, as with most things. I found it very complicated, and for me, it didn't work long-term.

I have developed my own approach to calorie counting. This is a personal system, not backed up by scientific research. I grade the calories in food, for reasons I will outline. My system is pretty simple:

- **FACE VALUE CALORIES:** Fresh, natural food calories are at face value. In fact, if you eat a fresh food diet, you do not need to concern yourself with calorie counting.

- **CALORIES x1.5:** Food that has added sugar, which is not the primary ingredient, I multiply those calories by 1.5. For example, let's look at a tin of soup. It has sugar added but it's not a sweet food, so I apply a 50% calorie tariff.

- **CALORIES X2:** Food with high added sugars, like biscuits and cakes, I double in value. So a chocolate bar that says 400 calories per bar, I class as double calories, so it is 800 calories.

- **CALORIES X3:** Pointless calories, like alcohol, I triple. A pint of lager has 180 calories, but they are really empty calories, so I multiply that by 3, and therefore, it has the equivalent of 540 calories in my system.

It is just my personal approach, but as I said, if you are counting calories, you are genuinely wasting your time. It doesn't work. It is a completely flawed system. All calories are not equal and I will explain why later.

Food labelling, in my view, is completely ineffective and misleading, giving completely misleading information, deliberately so. It simply doesn't really tell the full story. There are three villains that shoulder most of the blame for making us fat and unhealthy, which I call the 'SSS' gang. These are:

- Sugar (refined sugar)
- Sugar Substitutes
- Saturated and Transfats

There are very few processed foods that do not contain at least one of these evils. You could add salt to the list but as it doesn't actually make you fat, so salt gets away with not being included. The nutritional value of processed food has detreated so much in the last 30 years to the point where many people are eating hardly any of the recommended daily amounts of essential daily nutrients needed by their body.

These three bad boys are found in massive quantities in processed food and they are making us fat and ill, yet we can't get enough of them. People are eating more than ever. We eat more and more of it, year after year, in quantities that are really bad for us, so much that it has resulted in the huge rise in obesity and related diseases. Processed foods are chemically optimised to get us hooked and keep us addicted. Sugar, artificial sweeteners and manmade fats are the tools the manufacturers use to make us desire their product and sell more and more of the foods, which are bad for us.

Now, you may be thinking I am some tree hugging radical character from a commune, living off the land. Nothing could be further from the truth. I love food, all food, and believe me, if I could live off biscuits, chips, takeaways and Diet Coke, I would be in heaven. I love the taste of those foods. I get so much pleasure from them, too much pleasure.

Sadly though, there is a price to pay for this pleasure, as I have found out first hand. Weight gain, ill health (in my case two blood clots on the lung) and cravings, which lead to addiction. I have concluded that for every unit of pleasure you get from processed food, you get double the problems, as a result, at some time in the future. It's the basic cause and effect theory. This is a personal view but there is plenty, and I mean plenty, of scientific research to substantiate this contention.

If I was talking about the effects of smoking it would make perfect sense and you would not argue. The link is now universally accepted. Every cigarette you smoke today, giving you the instant gratification your cravings require, will contribute to health problems at some time in the future. The more you smoke, the more likely this is going to happen. Sure, everyone has heard of Uncle Charlie who smoked 60 a day until he was 96 and got knocked over by a bus. No rule is not 100%. The bus was probably the Monster Raving Looney Party battle bus, who get a handful of votes in elections, proving, like Uncle Charlie, that nothing has to add up to exactly 100% to be unanimous.

You can apply the same theory to taking drugs and excessive alcohol consumption. The fact that these can get you addicted and can cause serious health problems is a completely unchallenged statement. But that was not always the case. The debate about processed foods, or should I say what is in processed food, primarily sugars and fats, is at an earlier stage. The outcome will, ultimately, be the same and things will change - but at what cost to human health until it does?

Sugar is a substance that should sit alongside tobacco, drugs, and alcohol. It is equally highly addictive and dangerous to human health. In moderation, sugar is perfectly okay. The problem is that sugar is being consumed at toxic levels. If sugar consumption was equated to alcohol, most of us would be serious alcoholics. The consumption and prevalence of sugar in manufactured food is at levels the human race cannot sustain. Change must happen and change will happen, but you do not have the luxury of time.

Chapter 5
The big fat sugar problem

"If only a small fraction of what is already known about the effects of sugar were to be revealed in relation to any other material used as a food additive, that material would promptly be banned."
David Yudkin

Having made these bold statements about manufactured food being bad for us, and laying the blame squarely at the door of refined sugar, I will now substitute these claims. This is where it gets interesting or shocking, depending on your point of view. The issue of sugar and its effect on human health and nutrition merits a book all to itself. We will cover the basics, the headline facts only, but that is more than enough to make the point. The specific point is refined sugar is killing us. It is more addictive than cocaine and exceptionally bad for human health.

Sugar is a huge topic, which is starting to gather momentum. The wind of change is starting to blow, but it is no more than a breeze, stirring in some places, when it needs to be a Force 9 gale. People are starting to wake up to the fact, and it really is without question, that sugar is making us fat, unhealthy, and has gotten us all so addicted, we are eating ourselves into an early grave. We are eating sugar on an industrial scale; so much so, we are poisoning our own bodies.

It is important that we make a clear distinction between natural sugars and refined or processed sugar, known as sucrose, before we go any further. I am talking about manmade, refined sugars, sugars, which are added to foods, not sugars that are naturally present in fresh foods. These added sugars are also known as free sugars. The science is pretty boring (to most), but there are basically three naturally occurring sugars, Fructose, Glucose and Galactose. All other sugars are compounds (made of) one of these sugars.

Table sugar, which is the sugar with which we are most familiar, is made of glucose and fructose in equal quantities and known as Sucrose. The word 'sucrose' was first used in 1857 by the English chemist, William Miller, derived from the French sucre ('sugar') and the generic chemical suffix for sugars, ose. Sucrose is not naturally occurring; it is refined and a manmade compound. In 2013, it was estimated that 175 million metric tons of sucrose was produced worldwide. When I use the generic term sugar, I actually mean sucrose, the refined stuff.

There is also another version of refined sugar of which you need to be aware. This is a much cheaper version, called High Fructose Corn Syrup (HFCS), which is primarily used for food manufacturing, used widely in the USA, and is being consumed in ever increasing quantities worldwide.

Right, so that is clear. Refined sugar is the bad guy, because natural sugar consumed in fresh food is no problem at all. So here is a bit of basic biology. Scientists will find this a bit simplistic. That it might be, but it is accurate enough to illustrate that sugar is addictive, harmful and responsible for making us fat.

Sugar (sucrose), contains two molecules: it is one part glucose and one part fructose. Glucose is present in the human body; it is part of our metabolism. Our bodies produce it, and we have a constant supply of it in the bloodstream. Our body can deal with glucose, up to the point, where there becomes too much of it present.

Fructose, however, is not a natural part of our metabolism, and humans do not produce it. So back to the simple science again. Very few cells in the body can make use of fructose except liver cells. When we eat a lot of sugar, most of the fructose gets metabolized by the liver. There, it gets turned into fat, which is then secreted into the blood. So the more fructose you eat, the more your liver has to work. Do not worry about naturally occurring fructose in fruit. That is perfectly healthy and consumed at normal levels. You simply cannot consume enough fresh fruit at a time for it to become an issue.

Excess glucose in the body is toxic, so the body produces insulin in order to get the glucose out of the bloodstream and into the cells. If we didn't have insulin or it wasn't functioning correctly, blood glucose would reach toxic levels.

But, high consumption of fructose, the other half of sugar, can cause insulin resistance. Eating a lot of sugar chronically raises insulin levels in the blood, which selectively deposits energy from foods into fat cells, making us fat. When this gets out of control, you can develop type 2 diabetes. Unfortunately, the level of sugar we as a society are consuming is causing lots of health issues, and type 2 diabetes is right at the top of the list.

Type 2 diabetes is reaching epidemic proportions. Being overweight or obese is the main modifiable risk factor for type 2 diabetes. According to Public Health England:

"Obese adults are five times more likely to be diagnosed with diabetes than adults of a healthy weight. Currently 90% of adults with type 2 diabetes are overweight or obese. People with severe obesity are at greater risk of type 2 diabetes."

Basically, there is a direct link between obesity and diabetes. In many cases, type 2 diabetes is avoidable by following a healthy diet. Diabetes UK says not all obese and overweight people get diabetes, but you are far more likely to get it by eating too much sugar and by being overweight. As 90% of diagnosed type 2 diabetes patients are overweight, it is pretty conclusive.

Diabetes UK estimates that more than 1 in 16 people in the UK has diabetes (diagnosed or undiagnosed). That is around four million people. This has grown massively over the last 30 years. I am not a scientist, but I think only a fool would argue there is no link between rising sugar consumption and the rise in obesity, which in turn, leads to huge growth in harmful diseases, like type 2 diabetes.

In 2015, the NHS will carry out 7,000 limb amputations on patients with type 2 diabetes. 10% of the NHS budget is now taken by diabetes in the UK, around £9 billion. It is staggering, and the reality is, it is completely avoidable. Type 2 diabetes is caused, primarily, by sugar. If people with type 2 diabetes stopped eating sugar and only ate natural food, they would, in all likelihood, be free from diabetes within a few months. The more sugar you eat, the more chance you have of contracting type 2 diabetes. Here is a statistic that floored me when I heard it. 1 in 3 kids at the age of 11 are overweight or obese. Wow. What are parents doing, letting their kids get fat? If 33% of 11 year olds are overweight, the future looks gloomy to say the least.

Dr Robert Lustig, author of Fat Chance: The Bitter Truth about Sugar, argues cheap sugar is killing us. It has been added to your diet, and it is present in a wide range of foods, and too many of those foods where it doesn't need to be. When high-fat foods were blamed for making us overweight, manufacturers tumbled over each other to produce low-fat products. But, to make them palatable, they added sugar, causing much greater problems. When you add sugar to foods you cannot make them less sweet, as people won't like them as much, and they will buy less of it. Business just doesn't work that way!

Palatability is a buzz word in food manufacturing. Simply put, this is how appealing a food can be made to taste, which is the primary driver determining the success, in sales terms, of manufactured foods.

It is clear the drive for profit has prioritised palatability over the nutritional benefit of food. Sugar hits our 'sweet spot', which gives us instant pleasure when we taste it, stimulating receptors in the brain. The more we have of it, the more we crave it. We crave it so much, we eat more of it; the more we eat of it, the more harmful it is for us. There we go again with the vicious cycle.

I said I will substantiate my calorie multiplication theory. Lustig argues counting calories is not the answer because 'a calorie is not a calorie'. The effect of a calorie in sugar is different from the effect of a calorie in lean protein meat. Added sugar is often disguised in food labelling under carbohydrates and a myriad of different names, from glucose to diastatic malt and dextrose. Confused, you should be, but I think that's the idea of food labelling! But there you go, a proper scientist backs up my calorie multiplier. Not all calories are of equal value, which calls in to question the calorie counting method of nutrition.

The National Diet and Nutrition Survey (2013) based on self-reported consumption found that in the UK, we consume 60g of added sugars daily from all sources. That is around 15 teaspoons a day. However, any research that relies on self-reporting is always, as a rule, underestimated. I have seen other estimates that show the UK average daily intake is around 20 teaspoons a day. The media has published figures as high as 40 teaspoons. In truth, there are no accurate figures. What we can say is, whatever the precise figure, we are eating sugar at unsustainable levels.

The World Health Organisation recommends limiting daily sugars to 5% of your total daily calories, which is equal to 6 teaspoons for an adult of normal body mass index (BMI). Average consumption is way over what is recommended as being good for us. That is the root cause of obesity. Sugar in our food is the number one factor that can be directly linked to the world obesity epidemic.

The link between sugar in our diet and obesity is without question. But this, amazingly, has not long been the case. In the 1980's, the government issued guidelines to eat a low fat diet, putting the blame for making us fat firmly at the door of fat and carbohydrates. We became obsessed with a low fat diet. Foods labelled low in fat contained much higher levels of sugar. Yet, grouping all fats together is grossly misleading. Not all fat is bad for you, but there are some types of fats, yes you guessed it, the manufactured modified ones, which are bad for you, very bad. We will look at these in detail later, but compared to fat, sugar is much worse.

David Yudkin is the author of Pure White and Deadly. It is a fascinating read and an eye opener. Something millions of people take for granted is the source of so much misery. Once you have read this book, you will struggle to see the difference between tobacco and sugar.

He claims: "All human nutritional needs can be met in full without having to take a single spoonful of white brown or raw sugar."

We take it because we like it, but do we like it or are we actually addicted to it? More on that later! But he makes a statement, which when I first read it, being the first book I had read about sugar, I thought 'yeah, right'. But I have to say, the more I learn, the more I agree.

Yudkin says: *"If only a small fraction of what is already known about the effects of sugar were to be revealed in relation to any other material used as a food additive, that material would promptly be banned."*

According to the experts, excess consumption of added sugars is responsible for diseases that collectively kill millions of people per year worldwide. As well as diabetes, elevated insulin levels caused by excess sugar consumption could be fuelling a large increase in certain types of cancers, including breast and colon cancer. Sugar lowers your white blood cell count, reducing your immune system from everyday diseases.

We have not yet mentioned the most obvious issues linked to obesity, heart diseases, and strokes. Coronary heart disease (CHD) is the leading cause of death both in the UK and worldwide. It is responsible for more than 73,000 deaths in the UK each year. About 1 in 6 men and 1 in 10 women die from CHD. There is a direct link between sugar consumption and heart disease. A US study shows those with the highest sugar intake have a four-fold increase in their risk of heart attacks, compared to those with the lowest intakes. Fats have been unfairly blamed for many years. Some fats are actually really good for you, such as omega-3 fats, nuts, and olive oil, which were proven to reduce heart attack risk by more than 30% in a recent study. We have been given the wrong advice for years and look at the result. People are just getting fatter; it's actually scary! You can thank sugar for most of it, and the fact is that people are blissfully unaware of how much sugar they actually eat.

In 1915, it was estimated the average person consumed 5 kg of sugar every year. In 2015, that figure is likely to be close to 60 kg. It is quite clear we have a sugar based diet built around manufactured and processed food. We may be well fed, but as a society, we are undernourished.

The growth of sugar has hugely increased over the last 30 to 40 years as we moved away from a diet based around fresh fruit, veg and meat to one centred around manufactured high sugar food. I am sure we could correlate the move away from local grocers and butchers to supermarkets. We are living in a market where discount retailing is flourishing. You get what you pay for, I was always told, and the cheaper something gets, a decrease in quality usually follows. I wonder if the less you pay, the higher the sugar content becomes?

It is unrealistic to cut sugar out of your diet altogether, but as Lustig says, sugar is being consumed at levels that are toxic to the body. If your sugar intake is managed correctly, then you can enjoy some sugar in your diet and stay healthy. But right now, we are eating far too much, and most of us have actually have no idea just how much or where it is coming from.

A lot of the sugar we eat is under the radar. Food labelling needs a complete overhaul, and one of the important changes needs to be for labels to state the amount of 'free sugars' added to food. The government is advising us to regulate our sugar intake, but they need to make it possible for us to do so, easily. After all, you can't manage what you can't measure!

The only sugars that are excluded from the definition of 'free sugars' are those found naturally in whole fruit and vegetables and in milk. There is no evidence to suggest these natural sugars are associated with any harmful effects, but processed sugar is, without doubt, consumed in high volumes, is exceedingly harmful to the human body and mind.

No added sugar should mean just that, in all forms. I would like to see a traffic light system, green for no added sugar, orange for foods with a moderate level of added sugar, under the daily recommended level per serving, and red for foods with added sugars that exceed the daily suggested amount per day. This would make sugar management easier. Right now, it is almost impossible for people to comprehend.

The UK government recommends free or added sugars shouldn't make up more than 5% of the energy (calories) you get from food and drink each day. That's a maximum of 30g of added sugar a day for adults, which is roughly seven sugar cubes. Children should have less – no more than 19g a day for children aged 4 to 6 years old (five sugar cubes), and no more than 24g (six sugar cubes) for children aged 7 to 10 years old.

All well and good, but without the ability to monitor intake through processed food, people simply cannot manage their sugar consumption levels.

I strongly believe a labelling system should be introduced, showing the amount of added 'free sugars' to food in all forms. People who drink lots and get ill or who smoke loads and get ill only have themselves to blame, but sugar is so hidden that people are consuming so much sugar they do not know about, it is scandalous. The accepted unit is teaspoons (4g), so a labelling system should show the number of teaspoons of added sugars in certain foods. The guessing game has to end and end now.

The problem to overcome with sugar reduction is that it has everyone hooked. Sugar is cheap, plentiful and tastes so nice. Right now, people do not have the right information to make a sugar choice. If people were sufficiently advised and informed, then they could make an informed decision. We live in a sugar saturated society. We are consuming sugar at levels so toxic to our bodies that it is killing us.

The task for governments is huge, and in all reality, it is a battle that will never be won. Not entirely but the great news is, you can save yourself. If you are overweight and cut out, or at least drastically cut down, your sugar intake you will lose weight. I can guarantee this will happen in 100% of cases. This is a pretty bold statement, but I would happily put money on it.

I have learned so much about sugar, the harm it does, and the effect on the body. I have read so much about it and I have been genuinely shocked by what I have discovered. Everyone I have advised to cut out sugar for 28 days all lost weight, up to a stone. The end result is a huge increase in health and wellbeing. Sugar is everywhere and foods you perceive as healthy are not always what they seem.

Eating salads is a great example. There is no sugar in a salad, but add a dressing, even a 'low calorie' one, and it is laced with sugar. McDonalds is a great example; get a healthy salad, add a dressing, and it is healthy no more. I once checked the MacDonald's website, and a chicken Caesar salad with dressing and croutons contained 425 calories and 21.4g of fat, compared with the 253 calories and 7.7g of fat in their standard hamburger. Really healthy!

My policy now is to avoid sugar as much as possible and will be for the rest of my life. The reality is, you can't avoid sugar altogether, unless you exclusively eat real fresh food. The recommended daily sugar intake is 30g of sugar a day. To put this into context, a can of Coke (not Diet Coke) contains 35g of sugar. The daily advised amount blown out of the water in one can. Here is a list (published in the Daily Mail) of other popular snacks:

- Cadbury's Dairy Milk (45g bar) - 25g of sugar, the equivalent to five cubes
- Two McVitie's Digestive Biscuits (31g) - 5g of sugar, or one cube
- Muller Light yoghurt (175g) - 12.4g of sugar, or just over two cubes
- McDonald's Strawberry Milkshake - 62g of sugar, or 12 cubes
- Galaxy Minstrels (42g bag) - 28.9 of sugar, or six cubes
- Cadbury Twirl (two finger bar) - 24g of sugar, or five cubes
- Kit Kat Chunky - 23.7g of sugar, or four cubes
- Fruit Pastilles (seven sweets) - 15g of sugar, or three cubes

Sugar is also present in high quantities in unexpected foods. Salad dressings, cereal bars, yoghurts, sauces, you name it, and sugar is probably in it! Perhaps the area sugar consumption is at its highest is soft drinks. Fizzy drinks contain a huge amount of sugar, so do cordials and processed fruit juices.

Shockingly, children are consuming massive amounts of these drinks. Tooth decay in children is at an all-time high as is child obesity. I agree with the contention we are consuming sugar at toxic levels.

Frighteningly though, we are doing the same to our children. Beer and wine similarly contains huge amounts of sugar. The best thing you can do is drink nothing but water, until you hit your target weight at least. More about that in due course.

The labelling of food simply has to change. There is a great old saying, 'Bullshit Baffles Brains'. It seems to me this is what the labels on processed foods are designed to do. Sugar content has to be prominently displayed. This should become law if the obesity crisis is ever going to be tackled.

Sugar is like alcohol. In moderation, it is perfectly fine, but drink too much and you will do yourself long-term harm. Sadly, we are consuming sugar in the amounts that a chronic alcoholic would drink. Unfortunately, unlike alcohol and tobacco, we don't know how much we are taking on board. The tide is very slowly turning, but it needs to be much quicker. We need to become much more sugar savvy for the good of our health and waistline.

Why sugar makes us eat more

Time for some more high school biology to explain why consuming sugar actually makes us eat more. The fructose found in refined sugar makes the brain leptin resistant, which means the brain doesn't realise that there is stored fat in the body, so it acts and thinks like it is starving. This causes a powerful leptin-induced biochemical drive to keep eating even when we don't need to. In a nutshell, sugar takes the brakes off your appetite suppression systems.

Leptin, there is a new word. Leptin is released by fat cells. The bigger the fat cells, the more leptin they release, which acts like a signal to your brain to determine how much fat it has stored away. So if the brain knew you had plenty stored round the middle, it would use that before signalling you to eat again. The problem is the high levels of sugar we are consuming has broken this mechanism. The brain thinks you are starving and makes us eat more and burn less. When in fact, the opposite is true.

This explains why people fail at dieting. Your system is not working right and your basic survival instinct kicks in. The brain thinks you are starving and goes to Defcon 5, craving food and lots of it, so you eat. The result is, we get even fatter. Put in the most basic of terms, sugar stops your internal food regulation system from doing its job. That is why cutting out sugar is the easiest way to lose weight or essential for effective weight loss.

You should be starting to get the picture now. Sugar is making you fatter. Is sugar toxic? I think we can safely say our body is not designed to run very well on high levels of it, and we are clearly eating way too much of it.

So in view of all that information, we should just stop eating sugar. What's the problem? Well, unfortunately, there is a rather large obstacle to kicking the sugar habit.

Why we crave sugar

Wait, there is yet more bad news. For something so sweet, sugar leaves a bitter taste. Sugar has negative psychological effects on you, as well as the physiological problems detailed above. Sugar has a powerful effect on the reward system in the brain in the same way that leads to drug and tobacco addiction. Sugar activates powerful reward-seeking behaviour that can drive overeating. The more we eat, the more we crave it. Sugar is a highly addictive substance.

I cannot believe I actually wrote that sentence, but I have read so much about sugar and its effects, I am becoming dangerously close to sounding like a sugar militant. I have personally become much more determined to stop eating sugar for good. It really is wicked stuff. You cannot avoid it totally, but in trying to avoid it completely, you might just stay under the advised daily limit.

One of the first things I learned when I set out on my personal journey was that the human brain is hard wired to give us instant gratification. Dr Steve Peters, in his book, *The Chimp Paradox*, which was life changing for me, determined the brain is made of three elements: the human (you), the computer (processor and memory bank), and the chimp.

The chimp is irrational and driven by emotion and is motivated by pleasure. It has a very short term view and drives you to fulfil the pleasure you crave. Dr Peters argues that this drive is difficult to resist, because your chimp is five times more powerful than you, the human part of your brain.

Now note I deliberately used the word difficult, rather than impossible, to resist. We can manage our cravings and our drive for instant gratification. This is one of the cornerstones of the Freshplan and the Freshplan Mindset. But left unmanaged, you will constantly succumb to these desires to the point where you become addicted. Whether the addiction is to food or the sugar in food is a moot point. It is a problem we need to address to shift the pounds.

Sugar is addictive, because it hits a sweet spot (pardon the pun) in the brain. I recently watched a film, called *That Sugar Film*, where the presenter meets a food expert, called Howard Moskowitz. He says in the 1970's, he identified that everyone had a 'bliss point' for sugar. This is the amount of sugar we can eat before we think something is too sweet and tips us over the edge.

I used to sit in a restaurant, devouring a rich pudding and my wife would say, yuck, too sweet for me. Clearly, my bliss point is further up the scale than hers. Mind you, so was my waistline! The bliss point theory is applied to so many manufactured foods, including those that are perceived to be savoury, like pasta sauces, salad dressings, soups, you name it. It has a bliss point.

Food companies design foods for palatability or how desirable it is to the brain. They are looking for the optimal bliss point of food. My view is this is the primary driver in food manufacturing because it keeps you coming back for more and makes them big profits. Nutritional values seem to be a secondary consideration. The food industry will no doubt disagree, but if this was not the case, why would they use sugar in savoury foods like soup or in a salad dressing?

There is a perception that if food tastes really good, then it must surely have a high nutritional value. This is far from the case. I contend that the food industry is more concerned about hitting your sweet spot. The desirable qualities take precedent over nutritional concerns as far as the majority of manufactured food is concerned. There are exceptions of course, but sadly, they are in the minority.

The modern day diet is processed food based, with sugar being added in huge quantities, leading to toxic sugar consumption. The evidence is overwhelming. The calories in sucrose are empty calories. Having removed as much sucrose from my diet as it is possible to do, a life without sucrose is a much better one. David Yudkin pulls no punches, he says sugar is pure, white and deadly and we are eating it at toxic levels.

As I said at the start of this chapter, the subject of sugar and its effects is worthy of a whole book of its own. But I hope you have registered the key points:

- **Sugar occurs naturally in fresh food and milk, table sugar is sucrose**
- **Sucrose is manufactured, and is 1 part glucose and 1 part fructose**
- **The high consumption of fructose in sugar is responsible for many undesirable effects in the human body**
- **Sugar makes us fat and causes us to eat more**
- **Our brain craves sugar and is used in a wide range of manufactured food for this reason**
- **Our diet is processed based, and we are consuming toxic levels of sugar**
- **Cut out sugar and you will lose weight.**

Maybe you will agree now that not all calories are equal, and sugar is something you should cut out or seriously cut back on.

Sugar substitutes are not the answer

There have been many types of sugar substitutes developed, chemically produced to taste like sugar, but with no calories. For those of us who have been diet conscious, foods marketed as sugar free are appealing and can taste just as good. All the pleasure without the consequences. Think again. Diet cola is a great example; diet cola has almost no calories, yet tastes very sweet. As I said earlier, I was personally addicted to Diet Coke. I only drank Diet Coke; no other brand tasted the same. I was drinking five or six cans a day, sometimes more. Diet Coke contains Aspartame, which is an artificial sweetener. It also contains caffeine (there is a caffeine free version), which is also harmful in excessive quantities.

Though there is plenty of discussion as to whether artificial sweeteners are safe, having suffered serious health problems due to excessively consuming it, I advise, without hesitation, that you do not consume it, and if you do, make it very occasionally. This is a controversial issue, and the scientific answer is there is no categorical evidence to say sugar substitutes are safe, nor any to categorically prove it isn't.

The NHS website advises that in our digestion, Aspartame is quickly and completely broken down into by-products – including phenylalanine, aspartic acid and methanol – which then enter our system through normal routes. Hardly any aspartame enters the bloodstream. David Yudkin makes a valid point that any study that feeds excessive amounts of anything is likely to have negative outcomes on a living entity. I fully accept that point but I am living proof that excessive consumption is very bad for the human body.

In April 2015, Pepsi announced that it was dropping Aspartame as an artificial sweetener. They will now use Splenda, but for my mind, it is best to avoid diet drinks altogether. There is such a huge tide of negative health risks associated with it, why take the risk? I would make one observation. If something has no calories, then by definition, it offers us no nutritional value. But the fact there are no calories in sweeteners actually causes you to eat more sweet food and is the reason they should be avoided.

Here is some more science. Artificial sweeteners have been found to trigger enhanced activity within your brain's pleasure centres, the area that make you crave sugar, but as they provide less actual satisfaction, (they have no calories to burn) they lead you to crave more sweet foods.

Your brain gets the sweetness hit, but it doesn't find any calories to burn so the process is incomplete, so it drives you harder to satisfy its cravings. Therefore, you actually crave more sweet things by drinking artificial sweeteners. Your cravings go into overdrive.

This is what happened to me. Though I drank vast quantities of Diet Coke, with no calories in it, I craved more and got fatter by eating more sweet foods. My personal preference was biscuits. It is a vicious circle. That is a term we encounter a lot in relation to food and dieting. A vicious circle is exactly what it is!

The most important advice in this book:

If you take nothing else from this book, cut back on your sugar consumption, now. Become sugar aware. If you only do one thing, stop drinking all manufactured soft drinks. They have no nutritional value whatsoever and contain huge amounts of sugar. Do not drink diet soft drinks either. Fizzy drinks, sodas, cordials, fruit juices, diet drinks (especially diet drinks), everything, just cut them out of your diet forever. They serve one purpose, to make you fat!

Chapter 6
Saturated and transfats are really bad for us too!

For many years, in fact for the last 25 years, the official advice was to follow a low fat diet. Fats were seen as the big villain in the battle of the bulge, but in eating less fat we ate more sugar. The problem is not just the huge issues caused by sugar but also that some fats are actually good for you! Guess what it boils down to yet again. Natural fats are mainly good for you; manmade fats are mainly bad for you!

So yet again, there is a theme emerging. Anything that appears naturally in food and is unprocessed is good for you, or at least not very harmful, but when the food industry gets involved and manufactures food, it turns out to be bad for you!

So let's start at the beginning once again. Back to the high school biology. Or is it chemistry? Let's settle on calling it the science of fat. Again, if you have a degree in this, then you will no doubt scoff at the lack of detail, but as someone wanting to be healthy, the headline version is more than enough. So in simple terms:

There are four main types of fats that make up the fat in food:

Healthy fats are unsaturated fat, which consist of two types, **Monounsaturated and Polyunsaturated fats**. You may have heard of Omega-3 and Omega-6 fat. These are healthy fats. In fact, they are exceptionally good for you, in the right quantities.

Unhealthy fats are **Saturated and Transfats**. These are, without a doubt, bad for you. And guess what? These are the ones most widely used in processed food manufacture. Saturated fats are found in high quantities in processed meats, like sausages, ham, burgers. Fatty meat. Hard cheeses including cheddar. Whole milk and cream. Butter, lard, ghee, suet, palm oil and coconut oil. Transfats are mainly found in fried foods, takeaways, and snacks, like biscuits, cakes or pastries. Hard margarines.

Some fats are found in foods from plants and animals and are known as dietary fat. **Dietary fat** is a macronutrient that provides energy for your body. Fat is essential to your health because it supports a number of your body's functions. Some vitamins, for instance, must have fat to dissolve and nourish your body. So like sugar, there is some naturally occurring fat in natural food but this is perfectly OK and is indeed a requirement to make your digestive system work properly.

Eating a fresh food based diet, and one where you avoid processed food as much as you can, will cause you no problems whatsoever. The notion that all fat is bad simply is not true. In fact, some natural fat is exceptionally good for you. Omega-3 is top of that list.

Omega-3 comes from both animal and plant sources, most notably from krill and fish oil. Omega-3 supplements are big business but if you eat a healthy diet, you will get enough of this naturally and straight from the primary source is far better than manufactured supplements. There we go again. Fresh food is by far the best for you! There are different kinds of omega-3 fats but we do not need to go in to detail as it is perfectly correct to say all omega-3 fats are beneficial to your health. Primarily, they are really good news for your heart and cholesterol. Omega-3 also has a great impact on your brain health. It has been found to keep the dopamine levels in your brain high, increase neuronal growth in the frontal cortex of your brain, and increase cerebral circulation. Omega-3 is a really good fat.

Omega-6 fatty acids are also essential fatty acids. They are necessary for human health and must be consumed from food as the body can't make them. Just like omega-3, omega-6 plays a crucial role in brain function, as well as normal growth and development. They also help stimulate skin and hair growth, maintain bone health, regulate metabolism and maintain the reproductive system.

Before you start taking in as much omega 3 and 6 as you can, it is important to note that these should be consumed in equal measures. Unfortunately, because omega-6 comes from vegetable oils, the average diet, you know the one based on processed food, contains upwards of 10 times more omega-6 than omega-3. So right now, too many people are having too little omega-3 and far too much omega-6. The balance is unhealthy.

The whole issue of fats and health is immensely confusing, not least because there is conflicting advice. Traditionally animal and dairy fat has been seen as being really bad for you. There is now evidence pointing in the direction that it isn't animal fats causing our epidemic levels of heart disease, but vegetable oils. The term 'vegetable oil' actually refers to seed oil. You cannot actually get oil from a vegetable, just to complicate the issue even more.

There is great debate at the moment about saturated fats. For years, they were seen as unhealthy and we were advised to avoid them. Now, the smart money is on there being literally no reason to fear butter, meat or coconut oil, and these foods have been perfectly healthy all along. We were told to eat margarine and processed oils. Guess what, that may have been the wrong advice!

David Gillespie followed up his work on sugar with a book called *Toxic Oil*. He says butter consumption at the turn of the century was about 18 lbs per person per year, and the use of vegetable oils was non-existent. Cancer and heart disease were rare. Today, butter consumption is just above 4 lbs per person per year, while the use of vegetable oils and refined oils has soared.

David Gillespie puts it very succinctly, *"Modern biochemistry tells us that saturated fats and cholesterol are critical to the proper operation of the machine we walk around in. It also tells us that if we mess with the mix of fats we consume, we can significantly affect important systems in our bodies. When we look closely at how our bodies process and use fats, the truth about dietary fats becomes abundantly clear. The advice we have been and continue to be given is not just wrong, it is seriously endangering our health."*

What a surprise, folks! Food processing is taking healthy oils and making them unhealthy. This is done through a process called **hydrogenation** that is used to turn healthy oils into solids and prevent them from becoming rancid. This is the key. Most oil we eat is processed using this hydrogenation process. This makes healthy vegetable oils more like not-so-healthy transfats. On food label ingredient lists, this manufactured substance is typically listed as partially hydrogenated oil.

In simplistic terms, hydrogenation is a process by which vegetable oils are converted to solid fats simply by adding hydrogen atoms. Hydrogenation increases the shelf life and flavour stability of foods. As a result, it is found in a huge list of foods. This process of hydrogenation creates a transfat.

You name a processed food and it is likely to contain saturated or transfats, many contain both. Transfats are also produced when ordinary vegetable oils are heated to fry foods at very high temperatures and this is one reason takeaway foods are usually high in transfats.

You find transfats naturally in some dairy products and some meats. Though all transfats may be potentially unhealthy, no matter what their origin, if they are consumed at low levels, they are unlikely to have a significantly harmful effect.

Eating foods rich in transfats increases the amount of harmful cholesterol in the bloodstream and reduces the amount of beneficial cholesterol. Transfats create inflammation, which is linked to heart disease, stroke, diabetes, and other chronic conditions. They contribute to insulin resistance, which increases the risk of developing type 2 diabetes. Research from the Harvard School of Public Health found that transfats can harm health in even small amounts: for every 2% of calories from transfats consumed daily, the risk of heart disease rises by 23%.

The big, bad boys of the fat world are transfats. These are totally bad for you in just about every way. Whilst that may not be a scientific statement, it is not one a scientist would dispute.

I find the whole saturated fat debate baffling. There appears an answer to the question, are saturated fats OK to eat? If you want to lower your risk of disease, eat your Omega-3s but avoid the refined seed and vegetable oils. There is that word again, refined. Anything that gets refined, processed or manufactured appears to be harmful to humans. What a strange world this is. Humans make food for themselves that is really bad for them.

The use of oil in your diet should focus exclusively on naturally processed oils, like extra virgin oil. If like me, you have wondered what the difference between olive oil and extra virgin olive oil is. Well, it's actually simple. Olive oil is oil that is pressed from olives, the fruits of the olive tree. It is made by an easy process. You just press the olives (using an olive press) and the oil comes out. Some lower quality versions can be extracted using chemicals or even diluted with other cheaper oils. Extra Virgin Olive Oil means it is pure oil with nothing added.

There is enough debate to centre an entire book on fats and oils. But I have gleaned sticking to natural, fresh food is safe, and processed food is generally bad. Whether it relates to sugar or fat, processed food is basically full of really bad stuff that makes us fat and unwell. We live in a strange world, one where basically we are poisoning ourselves through what we eat and loving it.

Current UK government guidelines advise cutting down on all fats and replacing saturated fat with some unsaturated fat. Having read this, you may have read advice that is contradictory. The problem is there is no unanimously agreed advice. Transfats are undisputedly, appalling bad for you, but the debate over saturated fat continues.

The British Heart Foundation funded a study, which suggests there's not enough evidence to back the current UK government guidelines on the types of fat we eat. They think more research is needed before suggesting any major changes to healthy eating guidance. Whilst the scientists study and argue about the safety of processed fats in manufactured food, the one thing they all agree on is there is absolutely no risk and no harm to the human body or mind from eating nature's harvest. Fresh food is, without doubt, the best thing we can eat. There is no processed food that surpasses this in 100% of cases.

I may be screamed at for being a sensationalist but the food manufacturers have gotten us where they want us! We are hooked on the food they produce, and it makes big profits for them, because it is designed to be so desirable. In so doing, human nutritional requirements have, by and large, fallen by the wayside. Yet again, we can conclude that natural food is good for you, and as soon as the food manufacturing industry gets involved, it starts to get bad for you. The food we buy, processed food, really is not doing you any good. It is just about all bad for you. It's just a question of how bad a product actually is!

You are far better off avoiding manufactured food. If the fat doesn't get you, the sugar will. We have not mentioned salt, which is present in high levels in the food we buy. It is a preservative and high salt intake is bad for your blood pressure and increases the risk of heart disease. There is no wonder the world is fat and unhealthy.

Junk food is a term used for fast food, like burgers and takeaways. The reality is junk food appears to be any food that has been produced by humans and is best avoided altogether or consumed in the minimum possible quantities.

The media seems to have made the debate about the causes of major public health issues, such as heart disease, diabetes and obesity of fat versus sugar. The reality is they are both to blame and either or both consumed in high volumes, as is the case in our diet, is actually a toxic cocktail with the effects clear for all to see. The human race is getting fat, sick and dying younger. It is not a choice between cutting down fat or sugar.

Processed foods are making us fat, ill and addicted. Unless they are removed, or at least only consumed in small quantities from our diet, our bodies and mind will not function as they were designed and we will not be able to lose weight. You cannot lose weight eating processed food. It is almost impossible.

Chapter 7
Scientific proof that processed food is addictive

I have made the statement several times that processed food is addictive, because it is probably designed to be. This is actually backed by proper scientific research. If we accept that sugar is addictive, then it is a legitimate question to ask if sugar is deliberately added to so many foods specifically for this reason.

Dr Paul Kenny, a neuroscientist, has carried out research which shows how dangerous high fat and high sugar foods can be and suggests our brains may react in the same way to junk food as they do to drugs. "You lose control. It's the hallmark of addiction," claims Dr Kenny.

This assertion has been supported by several other studies. One of which was conducted by Harvard Medical School. They concluded that their findings "provide qualified support for the possibility of food addiction."

The study involved creating two milkshakes, one with a high and one with a low glycaemic index. The milkshakes were otherwise identical with similar calories and taste. The drinks were then given to 12 healthy, overweight men on different days and in random order. Four hours after the high glycaemic index shake, participants were hungrier than those who had consumed the low glycaemic index shake. No surprise there.

They then conducted brain scans on the subjects four hours later. They saw intense activation of the area of the brain that mediates pleasure eating, reward and craving (the dopaminergic, mesolimbic system for the scientists). The patterns seen are very similar to those found in people after the consumption of addictive substances, such as heroin and cocaine.

The brain is driving you to eat for reasons beyond physiological energy requirements. It is your drive to repeat the pleasure that is driving this type of eating. In a Connecticut College study in 2014, neuroscience students found that eating Oreos (a US biscuit brand) actually activated more neurons in the pleasure centres of rats' brains than consuming cocaine or morphine. Junk food junkies could be real, it seems.

You may be thinking this is crazy, biscuits and cocaine. The study compared how quickly the brain can become addicted to the effect they have on you, not how bad they actually are for you. If you compare the science that explains addiction, there are striking similarities between food and drug addiction. Addiction exerts a long and powerful influence on the brain that manifests in three distinct ways:

- **Craving for the object of addiction**
- **Loss of control over its use**
- **Continuing involvement with it despite adverse consequences**

If you are a cookie monster, like me, there is no question all three apply. The brain registers all pleasures in the same way drugs, winning money, sexual encounters and eating pleasurable food all release dopamine. Alcohol also as the same effect, but we will discuss the drink shortly. It is the dopamine that drives the addiction. The greater the pleasure, the more the brain produces.

Food manufacturers have known this for many years and are constantly researching ways to make food more attractive to our pleasure receptors. Author of *Sugar, Fat, Salt*, Michael Moss, recently wrote about ten components added to Doritos, specifically designed, to make them extremely tasty and difficult to resist. You quite often see 'improved new recipe' advertised on processed foods, such as crisps and drinks.

A cynic might say this actually means we have added more stuff to get you even more hooked. This strategy of processed food palatability is working. Consumers are hooked on sugar and fatty foods, most of which have limited or even zero nutritional value. People can't get enough of it. They know they are fat, and they know what is making them fat, yet the more they eat. It isn't logical, until you apply the addiction theory, then it makes perfect sense.

Sarah Leibowitz, a neurobiologist at Rockefeller University in New York City, has concluded eating fast food is indeed self-reinforcing. Her experiments show that exposure to fatty foods can quickly reconfigure the body's hormonal system to want yet more fat. So now it has been established that fat, as well as sugar, has addictive qualities.

Leibowitz found that it only takes one high-fat meal to stimulate this desire in the brain. What is all the more worrying is her statement that early exposure to fatty food could reconfigure children's bodies so they always choose fatty foods. Remember, 1 in 3 of the UK's 11 year olds is overweight.

Leibowitz found when she fed young rats a high-fat diet, they invariably became obese later in life. Her theory is an elevated level of fats, called triglycerides, in the bloodstream turns on genes that promote overeating.

This suggests that children fed kids' meals at fast-food restaurants are more likely to grow up to be burger loving long-term punters. Cynically looking at this, you may say giving away free toys to kids gets them young and for life. Surely they wouldn't be deliberately pursuing that as a strategy, would they? Maybe I have just become a cynical old so-and-so.

There is plenty more evidence to support the theory that manufactured food is addictive. John Hoebel, a psychologist at Princeton University (USA), recently showed rats fed a diet containing 25 percent sugar are thrown into a state of anxiety when the sugar is removed.

Their symptoms included chattering teeth and the shakes, which is similar, they say, to those seen in people withdrawing from nicotine or morphine. The study did not quantify what quantity of fat and sugar compares with a dose of a drug, such as heroin.

But Hoebel says, "Highly palatable foods and highly potent sexual stimuli are the only stimuli capable of activating the dopamine system with anywhere near the potency of addictive drugs."

You may argue that all his study actually proves is that rats like sugar but the weight of evidence is growing ever bigger. I am on board with this thinking, and indeed, my own experience of my battle with food over the last 30 years leaves no doubt that this is, by far, the most realistic explanation. Try cutting out all sugar from your diet for seven days. You will be surprised at what happens.

Ann Kelley, a neuroscientist at the University of Wisconsin Medical School, in the US, has uncovered evidence that eating sugar and fat-laced foods drives your brain to keep demanding you eat more and more. She found if rats' brains are overstimulated, they eat up to six times the amount of fat they normally consume. They also raise their intake of sweet, salty and alcohol-containing solutions, even when they are not hungry. Sound familiar?

Not only that, but they exhibited long-lasting changes in their brain chemistry, similar to those caused by extended use of morphine or heroin.

Ann Kelly concluded, "This says that mere exposure to pleasurable, tasty foods is enough to change gene expression, and that suggests you could be addicted to food!"

It makes perfect sense to me. I am incapable of eating just one biscuit. But have a banana and I do not have the desperate urge to immediately scoff another. I wonder, why? Do you think food may be manufactured with this in mind?

I have absolutely no doubt the only way to get thin, healthy and stay that way is to take back control of your brain function in relation to food and pursue a diet that your body requires to work correctly. It is blatantly apparent that a diet

predominately consisting of manmade foods, containing high levels of sugar and processed fats is, at best, detrimental and, at worst, toxic to the operation of the human body.

When I look back at what I used to eat and how I thought about food, it is no wonder I have been overweight and unhealthy for the best part of 30 of my 40-odd years on Earth.

How on earth can we get thin and healthy when the food we eat is so bad for us and [probably] deliberately designed to be so highly addictive? There is a huge, worldwide health crisis and almost everyone knows losing weight should be really easy, but it isn't, because our mind is working completely against us, which is exacerbated by the effect processed food has on us.

Key Point Summary, Processed Food:

- Processed food is the root cause of why we get fat. It contains excessive amounts of sugar and fats.
- Food manufacturers are more concerned with the palatability of food than its nutritional values.
- Sugar, as well as being high in calories, is also highly addictive. It prevents normal brain chemistry from correctly functioning, making us crave more.
- Sugar substitutes contain no calories but they trick the brain and, ultimately, lead to eating greater quantities of food.
- Food is designed to hit the bliss point in the brain and keep us wanting more. Research has shown sugar to be as addictive as tobacco

and drugs. This is why people ultimately fail at dieting.
- Natural fresh sugars, fats and food, in general, are not harmful to the human body or mind.

Part One:

THE FRESHPLAN MINDSET

Stop Failing, Start Losing!

Chapter 8

Willpower doesn't work: The dieter's negative mindset

You need to transform yourself from a failure into a loser. Of course, I mean a weight loser! When you start a diet, it tells you what to eat and simply apply willpower to see it through. That sounds so easy.

After all, we have complete control of our actions, don't we? Not quite. All it takes is willpower! Such a simple phrase but with 85% of dieters failing, something isn't working. Willpower is not enough because you face a constant battle in your mind and without the correct training, it is one you will lose time and time again. We fail at dieting because we fail at willpower. We fail at willpower because we do not know how to manage our decision-making patterns. The Freshplan gives you the gift of the POWER to say NO.

What is willpower anyway?

It is a word we often hear when it comes to losing weight. In fact, it is the key element to every diet and weight loss plan ever produced. But what does it mean? What the hell is willpower? They, the diet clubs and diet authors, tell you all you need is to follow their diet and a good dose of willpower, job done, easy as that. If you want it enough, you will do it, or so they keep saying. Well, I wanted to lose weight for years but I wanted biscuits more, in that moment anyway. I never managed to stick to any diet and the weight kept coming back and increasing.

I suspect this is a familiar story for many. The diet industry profits from it. It is a stand-off; dieters blame the diet for their failure, and the diets blame the people for not having the willpower to stick to the plan. Instead of addressing the key point of why so many people do not succeed, the endless cycle goes on.

In very basic terms, it sounds so simple. You decide what goes in your mouth, follow the plan and the weight falls off, and it should be that easy, but as everyone knows, it isn't. Simple it may be, but humans are complex beings. To succeed at dieting, you first need to have the tools to master willpower. You have to conquer the issues causing you to be a habitual failure. There is no one to blame, other than yourself. It all goes on in your head and that is where changes need to be made.

Without getting your mindset right, you will continue to live in the vicious circle of attempting, failing and frustration. If you do not address the willpower problem, you may as well save yourself the upset and not diet at all. I see many really overweight people in restaurants shovelling in fatty food. They have given up. There is probably some truth, on one level at least, in the saying that fat people are happy. They have at least accepted it and are free from the self-hatred that follows failing on yet another diet. But they will never be truly happy. You can't be fat and truly happy. It's a fact of being human.

I spent 30 years trapped in the vicious cycle of diet failure, never having control of my weight and believing I had no willpower. I realised that to ever lose weight, I had to become an expert in the art of willpower. I discovered the way we are wired. Our software, or mindware if you prefer, has default settings that virtually assure failure, every time.

If you look up willpower in the dictionary, it is succinctly defined as discipline and self-restraint. It sounds so simple. We would all like to think that we are in total control of every aspect of our lives, not just what we eat, what we do, what we say, how we act, everything.

The truth is, most of us, if not all, are not, and as far as weight management is concerned, the evidence is overwhelmingly conclusive. Most people are willpower failures when it comes to losing weight. Almost everyone I speak to say the same thing. They feel they are not in control of their thoughts, cravings and emotions in respect to food, giving in all too easily to impulse and switching far too easily into a state I have coined as 'sod-it' mode. We know it happens and just accept it.

'Sod-it' mode

'Sod-it' mode is the watered down term for what I call the point when you give in to your cravings. You can resist temptation no more; the goblin wins again. I see it in others now daily and recognise I very readily used to switch to sod-it mode. I actually used to say it, although using a slightly different word, as I finished off yet another packet of biscuits. When people have entered this state, they almost always say something similar to sod-it to justify out loud their action (of having cake, crisps, chocolate etc.) followed by some excuse. The ones I hear regularly are:

1. Life is too short, you only live once etc.
2. I will start dieting tomorrow, I will make up for it tomorrow etc.
3. I have had a stressful day, I have had a busy day, I deserve a treat etc.
4. I went to the gym today, I will go to the gym tomorrow, I have burnt a lot of calories today etc.

No doubt, you can add a few more to that list. It is a strange phenomenon that we feel the need to justify our failure to others, when really, it is to ourselves. New Year's resolutions are a great example. I don't know about you, but I had an annual ritual that included losing weight, joining a gym, and getting fit. You know the ones. I was lucky if I lasted a week. All I was doing was setting myself up to fail. One thing diet failures become very good at - excuses.

"He [or she] that is good for making excuses is seldom good for anything else." Benjamin Franklin

I have always thought I had the willpower. I would have sworn I had total control of my actions. But I was a superb excuse maker. I actually remember telling my partner I could lose weight if I wanted to. The reply I got was, "So why don't you want to lose weight then?"

This stopped me in my tracks somewhat. The thing with excuses is they crumble very easily when challenged. I actually wanted nothing more, and she knew it. But excuses are what we hide behind when we are overweight. We have nothing else. It is easier than admitting to failure. Any excuse will do, no matter how feeble.

I think diet clubs should do like Alcoholics Anonymous (at least they do in TV shows as I have never been) and open your first meeting with an admission:

"Hello, I'm Carl and I'm fat and a willpower failure."

That will probably have to be changed for political correctness. Replace the word fat with some more palatable term or remove it all together, but call it what you want. Fat is fat no matter how you spell it. We know we repeatedly fail to lose weight and have to find reasons for it, but really, they are just excuses and always feeble ones. Well, it's time to stop with the excuses, right now. Be honest. You don't actually believe them, and no one else actually cares. Face up to the fact that you want to lose weight but can't, because you fail at willpower. If you can admit that to yourself, you have taken another step forward.

I want you to say it out loud at least to yourself or preferably to someone close to you or write it down and email, text or whatever, as long as you do it. If you have been able to do that, then congratulations. You have made a huge breakthrough. It means any excuse you give in future for giving in will now be invalid. From now on, you are no longer going to fail at willpower or losing weight.

First, you need to understand why you are repeatedly unable to lose weight and how to stop failing and start winning. You can take total control of your willpower. It will be easy from here.

Research shows people, like me, who think they have the most willpower, are actually the most likely to give into temptation. The stronger you think you are, the weaker your resistance actually is. (The boffins term this as an inversely proportional relationship).

Of all the diets I have tried over the years, I now realise it is me that failed, not the diet. In fact, most of the diets out there will work if adhered to. But that two letter word, IF, is actually a very big word. In almost every instance, it was me that failed. I say almost, because there are some diets that are just downright ridiculous. The diet industry comes up with some extreme and ridiculous diet plans. I have realised this battle is won and lost in the mind, not on the plate.

I will say now that the diet plan you follow is almost never the problem. It is our willpower failure that causes us to fail at losing weight.

Kelly McGonigal, author of Maximum Willpower argues, "One thing the science of willpower makes clear is that everyone struggles in some way with temptation, addiction distraction and procrastination. These are not individual weaknesses that reveal our personal inadequacies- they are universal experiences and part of the human condition."

I don't particularly like the term 'willpower', because it is widely regarded as being easy, and giving in, saying yes when you want to say no, is weakness. I prefer to use the term MINDSET. I realised that to reach my personal goals, I had to completely change my mindset from one where I constantly gave in to temptation and desire to one where I was in control and the master of my own destiny. You have to change your entire mindset from one, which has been negative and expects to fail, to one that is positive, in control; the mindset of a winner, and you take success for granted.

I have used the term willpower deliberately because it is so closely linked and associated with weight loss. Willpower is one of those generic terms, like Hoover for vacuum cleaners and Coke for cola, so we will stick with it, but really, it is about your mindset as a whole. People who have better control of their attention, emotions and actions are better off almost any way you look at it. Your mindset is the key determinant of success or failure. It is within your power to adopt your mindset. Choose wisely young one, and the force will be with you.

Kelly McGonigal argues willpower is about harnessing the three powers of:

- **I will**
- **I won't**
- **I want**

You have to apply the right one at the right time to help you achieve your goals, and to succeed at self-control, you need to first know how to fail. Well, I knew how to fail, as I am sure you do too. I was an expert at failing, but I didn't know why I failed time after time. I repeated the same failings and felt like I was living in personal constant conflict with the greedy goblin within, the one I saw on the Sprite advert years ago. I recognised it, blamed it and had almost given up the fight when along came the London Olympics.

I am about to go off on a tangent, briefly, but bear with it. It will make sense, eventually. I was watching the Team GB Cycling Team clean up in the velodrome at London 2012. Almost a clean sweep of gold medals, total domination with eight golds for GB, they expected to win everything and I sensed some disappointment that they let a couple get away. What a radical transformation for a sport that GB traditionally was classed as minnows and the credit for this achievement lies firmly with Sir Dave Brailsford, head of GB Cycling.

You are probably expecting me to tell you to get on your bike and lose weight. No, stick with it a bit longer. I saw a great profile of Sir Dave Brailsford on TV, explaining how he deconstructed every aspect of the sport and rebuilt it, using a concept he described as the *"aggregation of marginal gains."*

His belief was if you improved every area related to cycling by just 1 percent, then all those small gains would add up to remarkable total improvement. I saw another interview in which Brailsford gave much of the credit for this success to Dr Steve Peters, who he said had totally transformed the mindset of the cyclists, turning them into winners.

Brailsford has described Dr Peters as 'a genius'. He turned a minority sport (in the UK) with a losing mindset into one, which believed it was unbeatable and indeed it became just that, totally unstoppable. Team Sky, who Brailsford and Peters worked with, won the Tour de France with Sir Bradley Wiggins, also in 2012, and has done it again, twice with Chris Froome (as at 2015). It is simply staggering what has happened to cycling in the UK. Other nations have openly accused team GB and Sky of cheating, using drugs but this falls in to the excuses for their own inability category, just like we do when we fail at dieting. Human nature in action, once again.

Stick with it; nearly there. By pure coincidence, in 2012, I saw a book on the shelf of Waterstones called *The Chimp Paradox* by the aforementioned Dr Steve Peters, now Professor Steve Peters. I paid my few quid and this book was a key moment in my life. It put things into focus and started a chain of events that led to the development of The Freshplan. I read everything I could, related to this subject, book after book and tested out many theories, adapting them for optimum success.

This brings us right back on track (no pun intended) and to the matter in hand. *The Chimp Paradox* is an excellent book, which you should buy and read. It covers all aspects of human behaviour and will be of benefit in other areas of your life. For me, it crystalized why I was not only having a constant personal inner battle and conflict with food, but it also explained why I always gave best to my greedy goblin within. I thought I was crackers until I read this book, but it seems I was right. We all have something living alongside us in our heads.

Psychologists have written about the two minds of the human brain and the battle we face between doing the right thing and the wrong thing, but few have offered the tools to conquer the conflict.

Some scientists believe we have two people living inside our mind. Two versions of us living in tandem, but in constant conflict. This would explain why one version acts on impulse and seeks immediate gratification with a sod-it approach to life, and the other attempts to control our urges and impulses in an attempt to achieve long-term goals. We can all easily identify with that.

Sometimes, we are the person who wants to lose weight, and sometimes we are the person who just wants to stuff their face. This is a classic paradox, the dieter's paradox, if you will. In *The Chimp Paradox*, Dr Peters introduces the Chimp model for mind management.

Though Psychology and the brain is extremely complex, this model makes it very straightforward to understand. The Chimp model states there are three basic elements to the human brain:

1. **The Computer Brain (parietal brain)**
2. **The Human Brain (frontal brain)**
3. **The Chimp Brain (limbic brain)**

We will use the simple terms, rather than the complicated ones. The computer brain is non analytical; it is where we store our memories and actions that we have learned. These are what Dr Peters call auto-pilots. Essentially, they are subconscious habits. These are things we do without thinking. Although they are pre-learned, they are not set in stone. Habits can be changed.

Where food is concerned, we often do things automatically, without realising. I call it the fat habit and we need to reprogram those to be healthy habits. The great news is that these healthy habits have a positive knock on effect to other aspects of your life, known as keystone habits. They play a crucial role in maintaining your wellbeing and we will discuss them in detail later.

The computer brain is constantly rewriting itself, sometimes for your benefit, sometimes not. However, we have the ability to take control of this process and instil positive and beneficial autopilots, or habits, into our subconscious. We don't need any hypnosis or trance-like state to do it either. I have tried that; it didn't work, and in my view it is unnecessary if it actually does work at all.

The human brain is in effect you. It is the person you want to be. It is the rational and calculating part of your brain, which looks long-term and is a strategic thinker, the sensible one, if you like. In terms of what you eat and other lifestyle choices, the human knows what is best for you and makes smart, sensible and objective decisions. The human brain has a plan for the future. The human brain is really good at dieting. The chimp brain is usually better at sabotaging those efforts, though, every bloody time!

The chimp brain behaves in completely the opposite manner to the human brain. The chimp brain acts on emotion and drives your desires and cravings. The chimp's aim, as well as keeping you safe, is to have a good time and get as much pleasure as it can. It is only concerned with instant gratification.

The chimp brain is the first one to send out thoughts, and when we have food cravings, they actually come from the chimp. The chimp part of the brain is five times more powerful than the human brain, which is the reason that we often give in to it. We are pushing against a force much stronger than us.

Within the chimp brain, I have narrowed it down further. Think of it as having a goblin living in the chimp part of your brain. The goblin is a 'good time Charlie', a greedy food monster. He (or she) is not concerned with anything other than living for right now. It seeks instant gratification. The goblin is not concerned about your long-term objectives. If the goblin desires something (like cake chocolate etc.), it will use pester power to get it. Once it has had one, it immediately wants more.

Have you ever had a biscuit and ended up eating the entire packet? I have many times. The goblin loves the taste, the sweetness and having had great pleasure from it, it wants more. The human brain knows this will lead to weight gain, it is unhealthy, and generally a bad idea. The goblin only wants to experience that pleasure again. Nothing else matters. The result is a conflict between the human and goblin, which lives in your chimp brain and with the chimp brain being more powerful without knowing how to manage it, the chimp brain usually always wins. The chimp brain is driven by emotion and emotions are often a trigger for eating. When the goblin wins, the human says sod-it and makes a feeble excuse. The more the goblin wins, the easier it is for it to do the same thing next time round.

The excuse is the human brain's justification for losing the battle. It is excusing failure. The goblin in your chimp brain is much like a dog. You are not responsible for the nature of the dog but you are certainly responsible for managing and training it to become well-behaved. If you have a dog and never train it, it will run riot and be very destructive; the chimp brain as a whole is much the same. Like a dog, if you train it, you can control it and you and the dog will both be happier for doing so.

So I was right all along. I do have a goblin in my head, and my goblin is a particularly greedy one. I have not slain the creature, but I call the shots now. It is very much under control. It is impossible to make that part of the brain inactive or remove all its power, because within the human brain, emotion is stronger than reason. This, therefore, is why willpower alone is ineffective and why 85% of dieters fail. So willpower alone is not enough to control the goblin. When you cannot control something, the best thing to do is to manage it.

Some scientists believe the human has one brain, but two minds. They are both us and we switch between the two. The key is to make the right decision, using the right part of the brain at the right time. When one part of the brain disagrees with the other, something has to give, one part of the brain has to win. The chimp brain usually wins but the human brain has the power to take control. By implementing the Fresh Mindset, we can take back the control.

The goblin has had its own way far too long. It has made you fat, it has manipulated you, taken control, lived it up and left you with the consequences of being overweight and unhealthy. The long-term impact of the goblin running the show is you will live less than you should and be less happy than you want to be. It is time for regime change, time for the human, i.e. you, to start running your own life.

The chimp brain isn't bad in terms that it is deliberately trying to kill you. It is there to keep you safe and make you happy. Your emotional responses to situations governed by the chimp brain are there to protect you, but in terms of food and weight loss, the goblin is quite unhelpful. As you embark on your weight loss plan, it will act like a petulant child and start pestering you like crazy. You have taken away its sweets, quite literally. No more cakes, biscuits, junk food, (add as applicable), but your goblin will demand them even harder from now on. It will start sending you messages that the food you are eating doesn't look good, smell good, or taste as good as the stuff you really want to eat. The goblin will pile the pressure on, using all the old reasoning like 'you deserve it' and 'what harm will one do?' Be ready.

Whenever you catch yourself having feelings, behaviours or thoughts you don't welcome or don't want, it means the chimp brain is at work. When you start craving sugar or junk food (again add as applicable to you), it is the goblin at work. For example, consider that you have been offered a piece of cake but you are trying to lose weight. Your human mind does not want to eat the cake, even though it looks nice and you know it is a nice cake.

The goblin will get to work and offer very persuasive reasons why you should eat the cake.

The goblin knows your weaknesses and how to get you to give in. If it doesn't get its own way, it will make you feel downbeat and make you think food, the wrong foods, will make you happy. It will strike when you are at your most vulnerable. When you are tired, feeling unwell, cold, upset, unhappy, angry, or whatever the problem, the goblin will prescribe food as a universal panacea. It will use the full repertoire of dirty tricks to sabotage your weight loss goals. It causes an emotional problem and comes up with a simple feel-good solution. The goblin is a master manipulator.

Self-sabotage is a phrase used in addiction therapy but let's not beat about the bush here. We are dealing with addiction. Psychologists broadly define self-sabotage as behaviour, which creates problems and interferes with long-standing goals. The most common self-sabotaging behaviours are procrastination, self-medication with drugs or alcohol, comfort eating and forms of self-harm.

Your goblin will make excuses for you to resolve your emotional state by eating. It will be very tempting and the goblin will make a persuasive case. You will feel good for a few minutes but will eventually feel worse if you give in. Self-sabotage always leads to self-loathing, and self-loathing only leads to one thing, total surrender. I am going to guess this sounds like a familiar pattern. The reality is, the goblin, which lives in your chimp brain, packs five times more clout than you, the human.

But all is not lost, in fact, far from it. The good news is, your chimp brain is not as smart as you, the human brain. It may have the brawn but you are the clever one and you can control it and get it working for you, not against you. Without doing this, you will be stuck with the typical dieter's mindset and the odds are stacked against success. In fact (here is my favourite statistic again), you have an 85% chance of failure, unless you manage your goblin.

DON'T WORRY YOU ARE NOT CRAZY!

Having read that you have two minds in one brain, you probably think you are crazy, or at least that I am. Well, you have no cause for concern. This is perfectly normal; everyone's brain functions this way. Although we are all different and have different individual traits, it is healthy to have conflicting rational and emotional elements.

If you are a psychologist, a psychiatrist or neuro-scientist, no doubt you will find this a far too simplified model but it is accurate enough for our purpose. There are three different aspects (human Chimp and Computer) of the brain. From a food, weight and fitness point of view, the model I am adopting is there is a greedy goblin that resides within your chimp brain. So we can define the three elements in our mind as:

- **YOU** - the true you, who wants to be thin, healthy and follow a strategy for a healthy, happy life
- **THE GREEDY GOBLIN** - lives in the moment, creates cravings and desire, using emotion and the promise of pleasure and enjoyment. Wants to eat lots of nice things

and leaves YOU to deal with the consequences

- **COMPUTER** - this is the memory bank that stores memories and runs the functions you undertake automatically, or subconsciously. It is constantly rewriting itself, often without you realising.

Having identified the problem, you are in a much stronger position than you have ever been. You can't fix a problem that has not been identified. Diagnosis is very often much more difficult than implementing a solution to any problem. This, my friends, is why you have been failing. Your mindset, through no fault of your own, has doomed you to failure. This is because it has had no management. With some simple changes, you can change this mindset to one that is extremely powerful and success will come easily.

You may be wondering why the hell the human brain works in this way. Again, the scientists will have ultra-complex and baffling explanations but the best explanation I can offer is that it is a result of evolution. Humans did not always live in a society where food was freely available and easy to come by. The cavemen didn't have a Waitrose round the corner. In fact, it is only very recently in the context of human existence that food has been freely available and we have ceased to use our basic hunter-gathering instincts. We can choose what to eat, when to eat and how much to eat.

Our chimp brains have evolved through evolution, and though in the context of the modern way of life it appears to be detrimental, in many ways, it actually has benefitted the human race. We have a fight or flight response mechanism driven, by the chimp brain, and an extremely strong survival instinct.

The human brain, as a whole, has led to the human race being the dominant species on the planet. This instinct is still there within us. Our brain drives us to eat as much as we can because in times gone by, there was not always food to eat. Enjoying nice things, things that tasted good, served us well, because in nature's food chain, there are foods that are good for us and foods that are bad for us; so bad, they can kill us.

Unfortunately, in this world we live in today, many of the basic human instincts and brain functionality has become obsolete. We have no need to eat everything we can get our hands on, all at once, as quickly as we can. There is no one going to come along and kill you to take it from you. It is not uncertain when you will find food again. This may sound rather silly but this is why your brain is behaving the way it does. It has evolved this way, but our way of life has radically changed.

When you look at it like this, it makes perfect sense. We, as a species, have gotten to this point in our evolution because of the magnificence of the human brain. Without these instincts, we wouldn't exist. This shows how wonderfully powerful and adaptable the brain is.

I have never spoken to anyone, who has weight issues, who hasn't identified the voice within, driving them to reach for the fridge or biscuit barrel. It is not some sort of mental illness; it is perfectly normal.

The chimp brain is not some dark side of your mind. It is good and bad. The brain, as a whole, is actually just a machine that can be reprogramed. After all, it is your brain and you are in control of it. Well, you will be when you learn to manage it.

The Freshplan gives you the tools to manage all elements of your brain and get them all working as one, in unison, to achieve your personal objectives.

You want to be thin, you will be thin, you want to stay thin and you can do that too. It is very easy once you have the right mindset. All you need now is your Freshplan to make it happen.

In terms of weight loss, the actual diet you follow becomes a secondary issue once you have the right mindset. As I stated previously, the basic principle of losing weight is as easy as it has always been. Eat fewer calories than you burn for a sustained period of time and bingo. Most diet plans will achieve this for you but whether or not you fail is based on if you have the right mindset. So let's make it happen!

Chapter 9

The Freshplan framework for success

The Freshplan follows a tried and tested approach, that of OST. Objectives, Strategy and Tactics. Broadly speaking, Objectives (and goals) define what you want to achieve. Strategy is what you will do to achieve them, and Tactics are the tools and tricks we will use in the implementation of our strategy to reach your objectives and goals.

There is a distinction to be made between Objectives, which are quantitative, i.e. measurable targets, such as weight and Goals, which are qualitative, i.e. personal to you, the reasons you are doing it and outcomes you hope to achieve. This is the framework for success we will follow.

In weight loss terms, this translates into a very simple approach. Simplicity is the key, every step of the way. Keep It Simple Stupid, or KISS, is something you should always adopt, because the more complicated something becomes, then so do your chances of success. The Freshplan Framework for success is simple:

- **Objectives - Set out your personal objectives and goals (they are not the same)**
- **Strategy - the diet / food plan you will follow in order to achieve them**

- **Tactics - use a set of effective tools to more effectively follow your strategy and achieve your goals and objectives.**

Successful people, teams and businesses have all planned to be successful. It very rarely, if at all, ever happens by accident. Certainly, you will not lose weight purely by chance. Without knowing where you want to get and what to do to get there is the difference between winning and losing, success and failure, and more pertinently, being fat or thin. You must plan to be and stay thin. It will not happen on its own. As you have probably found in the past, diets followed on their own or a strategy for weight loss is ineffective. A strategy without clear objectives and supporting tactics is simply not enough.

The Freshplan introduces you to a framework for success that has been tried and tested by the most successful people and organisations in the world in a wide spectrum of disciplines. If you can adopt the OST framework for winning gold medals, making millions in business and winning political elections, then losing a few pounds round your waist really should be a walk in the park, and it will be, quite literally. In his book, *Winners and How They Succeed*, Alistair Campbell, yes that Alistair Campbell, looks at this in detail.

It is a fascinating read and not at all political. Put aside any political bias you may have and give it a read. Whatever your thoughts about the author, this is a very good book on its own merits and a very worthwhile read.

"If you do not have a clear objective, you have no definition of winning. If you do not have a clear strategy, you have no chance of winning. And if all you have are tactics, you have no right to win."
Alistair Campbell

Campbell makes a really important point in this book, namely, strategy and tactics are all very well, but they are meaningless if the drive and discipline are not there to enact them. The Freshplan will give you the tools to maintain your discipline when things get tough. He also points out no matter how hard you work to stay on your own strategy, things happen all around you, all the time, which force you to adapt. This is very true. The Freshplan will ensure you keep on the path to success and achieve your weight loss objectives and personal goals.

Losing weight should, actually, be straightforward. You control what goes in your mouth, how much goes in your mouth and simply eating less and eating the right foods for a period of time will shed the excess weight stored by your body.

But in the real world, it is about so much more than that. Phrases, such as self-control, self-discipline and willpower, are bandied about all too easily when it comes to losing weight. But these are not just 'by the way, just add' elements of weight loss. They are the cornerstone of it. Added together, they add up to your mindset. Without the right mindset in place, you can't and won't ever succeed at losing weight and keeping it off. That is the key difference of The Freshplan.

The Freshplan transforms you from a 'NO I CAN'T, MINDSET' into a 'YES I CAN, AND YES I WILL' positive smarter thinker, who knows they will always succeed and never contemplates the notion of failure of any kind, ever again.

When I learnt that lesson after 30 years of hurt (which never stopped me from dreaming), success came and being the weight I want to be is now second nature to me. There is no longer a constant battle with weight for me. Peace has broken out, a fragile peace, but the entente cordiale resulting from implementation of the Freshplan will, as it has for me, change your life forever.

Creating your Freshplan

So you know what the causes of past failures have been, and therefore, you know what the potential pitfalls are as you embark on your personal Freshplan. Remember, you have ditched the excuses. You have made a statement admitting you have failed in the past, due to lack of willpower. Now it is time for you to make a change and implement a positive, winning Freshplan Mindset. This will achieve your objectives but to achieve them, you need to define them.

From this day forward, you must have total belief you will achieve your objectives. This is of primary importance. Success becomes the only possible outcome when you banish the notion of failure. You cannot change your past. Do not think of your past attempts at losing weight as failures and look upon them as finding ways that didn't work. You must learn to only visualise successful outcomes. The moment you contemplate failure, you open the door for it to walk through. From now on, success is in front of you. Do not look back, go forward and achieve success.

"If you believe you can do it, then everything else falls into place."
Floyd Mayweather

The chimp brain attaches great importance on successes, achievements and material possessions, whereas the human brain is more concerned with personal qualities. Yet again, the two brains have conflicting definitions of success.

However, by setting your objectives and planning the strategy you will adopt to achieve them, you can reward both the human and chimp brain. This will bring your chimp brain on side, working towards achieving a target. The goblin will still be pestering you for the wrong foods but it will be easier to manage as you work towards your target weight.

Your goals and objectives take on primary importance. They are the highest reward you can achieve and are far more important to you than a quickie with a chocolate bar. Focus on your goals and objectives from now on at all times. It is time for step one of the Freshplan.

The Freshplan has three elements:

1. **Where are you now? (Starting Point)**
2. **Where are you going? (Objectives and goals)**

3. How are you going to get there? (Strategy)

The Freshplan is a plan with a starting point, a set of objectives and goals with a strategy to get you there. This is where your journey begins. You have to decide where you want to go, and the Freshplan will show you how to get there, but first, it is time to dust off those scales and get a sharp dose of reality.

The journey begins – where are you now?

Your first job is to start a Freshplan Journal. This is a personal notebook of any size. I have an A5 ruled notebook and use a double page spread for every day. Use the left page to write down everything, and I mean everything, you eat and drink. Keeping a journal is a key part of the Freshplan and something you must do, every day. It is hugely effective in achieving success and reaching your personal targets.

Research suggests making a note of how much you eat can significantly help you lose weight. In one study, participants who kept daily food records lost twice as much weight as those who kept none.

I cannot overestimate the importance of your Freshplan journal. The object of creating a food diary is based on proven and successful research. You will use it to analyse what you are really eating. Food journaling has been shown to be a keystone habit that can make you healthier, happier and more productive.

Keystone habits lead to the development of multiple good habits. They have a knock-on effect in your life that produces a number of positive outcomes. They are small changes that lead to big differences. We will return to this subject shortly.

It is really important not only to write your journal but also to take the time to read what you have written regularly. The Freshplan journal will not only be a list of what you eat and drink but you will also use it to document successes and failures. Writing down your thoughts is critical to the Freshplan, but more about that later.

The first entry in the journal is to document where your journey starts, so you need to dust off those scales. I'm guessing you haven't used them much recently. If you are buying some scales, you may want to buy some modern digital ones that store your weight and link to a mobile app. They are quite expensive and not essential but the app will show your weight loss in fancy graphics.

Weigh yourself first thing in the morning and ideally naked or just in your underwear. As you record your progress, you must do so at the same time every day. There is no point in hiding from the truth. I have known people start a diet not knowing what they weighed because they were so scared of seeing their weight.

Similarly, I know people who over-inflated it, so it would appear they lost weight. When all is said and done, you might kid others but you will only be fooling yourself. The first steps are always the most painful ones, but it gets easier, one step at a time.

This is what you (ideally) need to measure on day 1:

- Your weight- the starting point for your weight loss (essential)
- Your measurements, waist, chest (essential)

You may also want to get the following information, which you can get from a health check at your local chemist or surgeon, but is not essential to the plan:

- Blood pressure
- Resting heart rate
- Cholesterol
- Blood sugar level

The key performance indicator is obviously your weight, but keeping a log of your measurements is also a good idea, because it is additionally motivating to see yourself shrinking. The medical data is also worthwhile, because you will not only see yourself getting lighter and smaller, but also healthier. The more you can see yourself achieving, the better it is for motivation and keeping your chimp brain on side and the goblin quiet.

You can now measure all your key vital signs yourself. My personal health indicators are a great source of satisfaction, and continuous monitoring and recording is highly motivating for me.

Indicator	Starting Point	Present Position
Weight:	19st 12lb	15st 10lb
Waist:	42 inches	36 inches
Chest:	52 inches	44 inches
Blood Pressure:	120/80	111/72

Resting Heart Rate:	74 bpm	48 bpm
Oxygen Saturation	98%	99%
Blood Sugar	'normal'	5.1
Cholesterol:	6.1	4.2

I have scales and a blood pressure monitor, which connect by Bluetooth and record the data to an app on my iPhone. I use Withings; they have a good app. They are quite expensive and not essential, but they keep a superb log of your data and show it in graphical form.

The level of data and storing it using these devices is superb. They are expensive, relatively, but in the great scheme of things, think of what you will save cutting back on luxury food and drink! They are a great investment. I take a readout once a week since it is quick and easy.

To measure heart rate and saturation, you can use a finger sensor, like the doctor would use. These are around £20 on Amazon. In my view, everyone should keep a close eye on their key health indicators. Ignorance is not bliss. It is so uplifting to objectively witness yourself getting lighter, healthier and fitter. Quantifying your success will uplift you.

Normal ranges for your health indicators:

- **Blood Pressure:** should normally be less than 120/80 mm Hg (less than 120 systolic AND less than 80 diastolic) for an adult age 20 or over. When getting your BP monitored externally, you can get an artificially high reading; this is called white coat syndrome. It is preferable to have home testing if this is the case.

- **Resting Heart Rate:** measure in beats per minute (BPM). A normal resting heart rate for adults ranges from 60 to 100 beats a minute. Generally, a lower heart rate at rest implies more efficient heart function and better cardiovascular fitness. For example, a well-trained athlete might have a normal resting heart rate closer to 40 beats a minute. Anything below 60 is a good indicator of physical fitness.

- **Oxygen Saturation:** or SATS is a term referring to the concentration of oxygen in the blood. It measures the percentage of hemoglobin binding sites in the bloodstream occupied by oxygen. Normal blood oxygen levels are considered 95-100 percent. If below 90, you should see a doctor immediately.

- **Blood Sugar Levels:** Normal blood glucose level in humans is about 4 mm (4 mmol/L or 72 mg/dL). When operating normally, the body restores blood sugar levels to a range of 4.4 to 6.1 mmol/L (82 to 110 mg/dL). Shortly after a meal the blood glucose level may rise temporarily up to 7.8 mmol/L (140 mg/dL). I check my blood sugar only once a month now.

- **Cholesterol:** a simple blood test used to determine the amount of bad cholesterol (low-density lipoprotein, or LDL), good cholesterol (high-density lipoprotein, or HDL) and triglycerides (other fatty substances) in your blood. You should have a level under 5.

I did not know how to monitor my own blood sugar when I started this. My doctor simply said I was within normal range. I have only recently discovered how to test it myself. You can buy, fairly cheaply, a home blood sugar monitor. I bought one for only £15 from Amazon. You prick your finger, drip blood on to a strip, and it gives you a reading. Simple really.

You can get your cholesterol tested at a pharmacy or even at your doctors. You can buy home cholesterol testing kits, which are a good indicator, but not as accurate as a proper medical assessment.

However, for your own use, these are perfectly adequate and are not expensive. If you show a high reading on the home kit, see a doctor. My doctor told me they like to see good news from patients and never think you are wasting their time. After all, prevention is better than cure.

You may wonder why there is no mention of BMI (body mass index). Well, health professionals will want to see me strung up for this, but I do not like BMI. It is a calculation based on the height and weight of a person to show the percentage of body fat in the body.

For me, personally, it has always been inaccurate to the point of being ludicrous. I think everyone knows the weight they should be. When I did that, I was 15 stone 10 and felt great. I could not be 10st 4lb; I am a big bloke with a big frame.

It is ridiculous to suggest I could and should lose a further 5 ½ stone. Even at the top end of that, 13 stone, would make me look gaunt and unhealthy. I look perfectly healthy, because I am perfectly healthy. I am training for a 10k run, an objective I have set myself to do in under an hour. I have never been fitter than I am today, but imagine how demotivating this would be for me if I didn't know to not waste my time and calculate it in the first place.

This is what I think. If you stand almost naked in front of a full length mirror, and you are genuinely happy with what you see, then that is your ideal weight. BMI, in my view, is far too generalised and simplistic. No two people are the same, and I believe it can be more unhelpful and destructive than positive. My advice is to forget BMI. But I am not just basing that on myself. There is some proper research to support my opinion. BMI is an inaccurate measure of body fat content that does not take into account muscle mass, bone density, overall body composition, and racial and sex differences say researchers from the Perelman School of Medicine, University of Pennsylvania. There you go; I am a case in point.

But there are plenty like me. Lifehacker.com has published an excellent illustration of this online. They show six people in the illustration who are all 5 feet 9 inches tall and weigh 12 stone 2 pounds (172 pounds in US-speak), which means they have the same BMI of 25.4. Enough said. Forget BMI, it will not serve you well.

So step on those scales, get it over and done with! At this point, you may be feeling depressed. Many people who are overweight haven't weighed themselves regularly, often not at all for years. I know, when I was overweight, I would avoid getting weighed at all costs, and if I was ever asked how heavy I was, I could feel my heart start racing.

I honestly didn't want to know and preferred blissful ignorance. But put your emotions aside. It is just a number. Look at it like this. The heavier you are, and the worse those numbers appear, the more weight you will lose, and the bigger success you will be once you have achieved your target. It is also the heaviest you will ever be.

You will never be heavier than you are today!

The good news is, this is now out of the way. The news will only get better from here. Every journey starts with the first step, and step 1 is the hardest step, but it is the biggest step. You may have been dreading it, but be honest. It wasn't that bad was it? You have a starting point in numbers. You know where you are and your starting point.

IMPORTANT

You are probably fired up and ready for the fight, highly motivated and ready to get started. You may be tempted to jump straight to the Freshplan Diet, but resist that temptation. Do not start until you have read everything. It is important you do not short cut the learning process.

SET YOUR OBJECTIVES AND GOALS- WHERE ARE YOU GOING?

The next job is to define your objectives and goals. Objectives and goals are not the same. Objectives are the numbers, your target weight, measurements, anything that can be measured on a scale. They are quantifiable objectives. Goals are much more subjective, what I term your personal feel-good factors, and you are the only barometer for these. You can't measure the feel-good factor, but you can record them in your Freshplan journal, and it is vital that you do this on a regular basis.

Let's start with setting your objectives, before we look at your goals. First question is the obvious one:

What is your target weight?

As I said earlier, you will probably know where you want to get. It doesn't have to be set in stone at this point, but it does need to be realistic. If I had set my target at the lower end of the BMI recommendation, it wouldn't have been achievable, and setting impossible targets is demotivating and pointless.

Having a plan with achievable objectives greatly increases your chances of success. If you want to be successful, you must not let the chimp brain and the greedy goblin interfere with your plans. Having a target that is not achievable is playing straight into their hands. Self-doubt will creep in, and the likelihood of entering into sod-it mode increases.

So set a weight that is achievable and realistic. Similarly, there is no point in setting a target that is too easy. I think everyone knows what weight they ideally want to be. So you can set your target weight and also easily calculate how much you have to lose.

You also know what size you want to end up. For example, I was a 42 waist and wanted to be a 36 waist. I was a 54 chest and wanted to be a 44. I am at a weight and size, no matter what the BMI calculator says, I am happy with. I am sure I could lose more, but I have a life to lead, and I am not going to become an athlete anytime soon. I have set a target I could achieve, but more importantly, one I can maintain with a happy weight-life balance.

You must remember this is not a one off project where you hit your target weight and then slip back into the old ways and pile it back on slowly or quickly. One of your mandatory goals is to get the weight off and keep it off for life. If you set your target weight too low, then maintaining it will be so hard, you will be unhappy and depressed. Set a realistic and healthy weight you want to be.

You can have as many health issues by being underweight and under nourished as you can being overweight. Once you have hit your target weight, you will set upper and lower thresholds, which you must not exceed. It is a long way from where you began, but one day, you may need to put a few pounds on to stay within your acceptable weight range. Only a small percentage of people who lose weight keep it off long-term.

My background is in racing, and I have seen jockeys maintain unhealthy weights for years on end. This is sad to see, and I know one former jockey, who became a depressed, moody, and angry person, battling to maintain his riding weight. He fell out with almost everyone and became a person, even he says, he hated. The day he retired from riding, everything changed. You would not call him overweight now, but he has gained almost two stone. Being underweight is harmful. Being underweight by design is a complete no-no.

The distinction between objectives and goals is not always as clear cut as I am describing, but the Freshplan draws clear lines. Objectives and goals are both targets, but are measured in different ways. Objectives are much easier. They are statements of facts. Goals are personal to you and drive your motivation.

If you read any book on management and strategic planning, you will come across the term SMART. This is an acronym to determine what your objectives should be:

- Specific
- Measurable
- Attainable
- Realistic
- Trackable

SMART applies perfectly here. Set your objectives accordingly. They have to be specific. No point in writing down to lose some weight or lose lots of weight.

Do not slip in to false hope syndrome by setting unrealistic expectations about the changes you want to make. It can become a vicious cycle if you fall victim to this, and you will fail every time if you set impossible objectives. The same applies to your personal goals.

Your Goals- What do you want to achieve?

Goals are much more subjective. They are specific to you and are what drives and motivates you. It is important to set these personal goals, but equally, it is important to keep the list short. The fewer goals you have, the easier they are to achieve. Focus is the keyword here. Keep the list short, but make them really important!

For me, I wanted to understand why I was so fat and unhealthy, and completely reverse that forever. I wanted to control my relationship with food and never go back to the person I was. I later set myself a goal of being able to buy a Reiss Suit, which are only sold to a 46 inch chest. To do this, I had to achieve my objective of being under 16 stone.

It can be as simple as you want it to be. If you achieve your target weight, you may be happy, and that may be enough. You must also resolve once you have achieved your target weight, you must never go back to your old ways. If you do not make this a goal, there is no point in losing weight in the first place. Your goals are for life, not just for now.

The goals you set can actually mean the difference between success and failure. Sensible and achievable goals will keep you focused and motivated. You are designing your own blueprint for change, and your goals are your personal Freshplan for a new happier and healthier life. When the going gets tough, your goals need to be very important to you to reinforce your motivation.

The one thing about change is it is inevitable. You are going to change as you get older, like it or not. It is a fact we cannot escape, so having some control over the nature of the changes you will experience is a positive thing.

A key point about the goals you set is to remember they are not a destination but a journey. By that, I mean, if you set a goal of feeling good about your body image, maybe a beach body that makes you a more confident person, then why on earth would you want to reach this and then let it go.

Your goals are not set in stone from day one. You can change them as you go. Indeed you will need to. Certainly, mine have changed. I achieved my first set of objectives, and I modified my goals, adding one of completing a 10k run in under an hour. In the above example of getting a beach body and body confidence, you will simply modify that goal to maintaining it permanently.

Not all weight-loss goals are helpful. Unrealistic and overly aggressive weight-loss goals can undermine your efforts. So write a simple list of what you want to personally achieve by losing weight. They will be specific to you, but your first Freshplan Journal may look something like this;

Date: *01/01/2014*
Current Weight: *19st 10lb*
Measurements: *Waist: 42inch Chest 52inch*

Resting Heart Rate: *69bpm*
Cholesterol: *6.1*
Carl Harris' Objectives:
Target Weight: *15st 10lb*
Weight Loss Target: *4st (56lb)*

Carl Harris' Goals:

- *To reach my target weight and maintain it for life.*
- *Have confidence to look in the mirror*
- *To be in control of what I eat and not give in to cravings*
- *To feel healthy, lower my health indicators into all normal range.*
- *To be able to wear a Reiss Suit.*

That is a very basic entry, which states where you are now, where you want to get, and what you personally want to achieve. The first goal is the only mandatory goal that everyone must set.

When setting personal goals, I like to implement the Gene Simmons principle. He is the lead singer of rock band KISS, which is an acronym for Keep It Simple Stupid. Do not over complicate the issue. Keep it simple for focus, which will help you achieve success.

Reading this book and the process of writing your goals and objectives is not enough to make things happen. You need to put in the work. The Freshplan will give you the tools to make sure you have the best possible chance of succeeding.

So now, we know where we are starting and where we want to get, we need a plan to get there as quickly and as easily as possible. This is where your Freshplan starts. Your goals and objectives are set, so let's go and achieve them.

Chapter 10
You have the power to say NO!

You have a starting point and stated destination, and your goals and objectives are set. Now you need to put a plan in place to get there. This is where the battle begins. You against the Goblin. The new you, one who expects to win and refuses to even contemplate failure. You want to succeed, the Goblin would like you to succeed too, but it isn't going to help you. In fact, it is going to do everything it can to make you look after its' own interests, which causes you to fail. After all, it has always won when you have gone up against it in the past, but this time, you are implementing the Freshplan Mindset, and you will succeed.

To achieve any objective, you need a plan. The Strategy you use to get there is the diet you choose. As I have previously stated, in many ways, the actual diet you adopt is secondary, because they nearly all work if you stick to them. Sticking to it is where things usually come unstuck, so to speak. So it is very much up to you what diet you follow. Of course, The Freshplan has a suggested strategy, The Freshplan Diet, which is highly effective, nutritious, and tastes good. It is, as many of the best solutions in life are, very simple to follow. I would recommend you give it a try, but it is your mindset and your ability to maintain the motivation and willpower to stick to a diet, which is the key determinant of success.

If you stick to your diet strategy, you will lose weight. The problem is when temptation comes calling. Unfortunately, you don't know when that will be. Remember, the greedy goblin is constantly seeking instant gratification. The goblin likes things that taste great. Having the enjoyment right now is more important to the goblin than achieving your goals and objectives. Having established the chimp brain is five times more powerful than the human brain, we need to employ smarter tactics in order to overcome your cravings and desires.

Your chimp brain has two primary motivations:

- To enjoy as much and as many pleasurable experiences as possible. This is the goblin's raison d'etre
- To avoid exertion and pain, as well as always looking to take the easy way.

I have developed a process to be employed when the goblin starts to step on the pester power pedal. There is no mistaking the cravings, and the more you deny the goblin, the louder it will scream. Previously, you would have eventually, or even immediately, given in and slipped all too easily in to sod-it mode. For too long, you have been enslaved by your cravings, and you have danced to the tune played by the goblin.

Now though, you have the **FRESHPLAN POWER** to manage your cravings and head off your goblin's attempt to sabotage your plan. When you have strong food cravings, you should go through the following five steps:

Pause
Objectives
Why & What If
Evaluate
Reinforce and Reaction

Before you take any action, whatsoever, you must go through this process methodically in your mind. It is not a long process. In fact, you can go through these five steps in a matter of seconds, if not under a second. The Freshplan Power Technique will give you conscious control of your actions, rather than instantly buckling capitulating and giving up on your objectives in favour of instant gratification. You have the POWER to control what goes into your mouth. When all is said and done, diet success boils down to controlling what you do and not putting it in your mouth.

You have a diet in place, and if you stick to it you will make it happen. Without this technique, impulse takes over, and you have given in almost without realising. You are going to replace impulse reactions with measured POWER decisions. When the cravings kick in, go through this process:

PAUSE - Press Pause Before You Make Any Decision.

The most powerful thing you can ever do is press pause. Imagine you have a pause button to stop everything, like you can on TV. This is a technique I now use in every aspect of my life. No action I take now is ever reactive. You need to stop being reactive and instinctive. The most successful people are proactive in their decision making. My Dad used to say nothing is gained by acting in haste, only a baby! It is all too easy to give in to your urges, but there are consequences for every action. You need to PAUSE and consider your action before you react.

I cannot stress enough the power of PAUSE. There are two primary advantages for Pressing Pause. First, it takes harmful decision making away from the subconscious. There are many repetitive behaviours, which you will do as part of your routine. Remove impulse decision making from your life, and you will always make smarter decisions.

There are many decisions made on autopilot, and you only realise after the event. For example, if you get home from work and instinctively pour yourself a glass of wine every night, because you have done this so frequently, it becomes normal behaviour.

You may often be several sips into your glass before you consciously recognise what you are doing. Often, you can't even remember the action of opening the bottle and pouring the wine. Pressing pause will stop this from happening on autopilot. You may ultimately choose to have a glass of wine, but you are doing it because you consciously decide to not because it is something you have programmed your subconscious to do as a matter of routine.

The second benefit is you are not susceptible to succumbing so easily to your cravings and urges for food. Before you give in and say 'sod-it', pressing PAUSE will strengthen your resolve. Think back to what you were taught as a child, the Green Cross Code. Stop, look and listen. This is a mantra that will serve you well in regard to your food choices. By pressing PAUSE, you are taking a stand and you already have more power over the goblin than ever before. You are asking the goblin to justify its request.

By pressing PAUSE, you are introducing awareness into your food decisions. Over 90% of our total decisions are made with little or no conscious effort and understanding why we made those decisions. This awareness around food choices is important. You must consciously participate in all food related decisions from now on.

OBJECTIVES - is this decision in line with your stated objectives?

You have already written down your objectives and your personal goals. You need to ask yourself if this action will contribute to achieving them, or is it in direct conflict with them. If the decision is in line with your objectives and part of the plan, then it is fine to go ahead, but the reality is, this is highly unlikely to be the case.

Clearly, if this is a decision about having a chocolate or cake (insert as required), then eating it will be counterproductive. The decision to say 'sod-it' and have just one or one piece (again insert as required) has now taken on greater significance. You are basically making a decision to go off the plan and break the diet. Is that what you want?

WHY? What is your Why and What If's Plans?

You are about to make a decision. But look beyond that few moments of pleasure you will experience. Why may be a small word, but it is a big question. You must ask yourself WHY?

- Why would you jeopardise all the work you have done so far?
- Why would you compromise your chances of success?
- Why do you want to go back to being the person you don't like being?
- Why would you want to trade the good feeling of achievement for the lows associated with failure?

You may want that pleasure of eating the object of your desire, but you will feel bad after eating it. You know you will regret making the wrong decision. You know full well that after the pleasure, comes the guilt. The pleasure lasts only a few moments; the guilt lasts a lot longer.

With a powerful 'why' you will find it easier to resist temptation. When faced with a craving, you must remind yourself of the reason you want to say no. These are your powerful personal goals. Giving in to your cravings on impulse is the easy way. By giving yourself time to do this, your self-control mechanism will kick in and help you avoid ruining your progress. Your goals are a higher reward for you than a quick sugar hit.

Of course, we are talking about eating just one biscuit or piece of chocolate, but it is not just one, is it? You know one leads to another; hence, what you see when you look in the mirror. You know full well what will happen. Ask yourself WHY you would want to put yourself through this.

You also know this is a natural process you go through, and your goblin will start to shout and pester louder and harder than ever before. You have a bigger reward waiting for you. When you start to see results, saying no does become easier.

Also, you will have a series of 'what if' responses ready. You may have experienced this before and even given in. Your journaling will help you here. 'What If' responses are your defences ready to scramble into action.

The one thing you know is your goblin cravings are not going to stop. Once a biscuit munching chocoholic, always a biscuit munching chocoholic! Be prepared with a range of responses to bring into play. If you have successfully encountered this scenario before, then think back to both the action you took and the feeling of achievement and superiority you felt. Your chimp brain likes to feel good and likes achievement, so offer a higher reward than the pleasure that will last only a few moments.

There is no magic panacea I can offer here, because as humans, we are all different. You will find what works best for you. With every no you say, the next one becomes easier. Now you have gathered all the facts....

EVALUATE - You have to justify your decision to yourself.

With all the facts and ramifications in place, you need to evaluate the best course of action. The request from the goblin is based on emotional triggers. Desire for pleasure is the key driver, but you need to change the nature of this decision from an emotionally driven one to an objective, rational one. When you evaluate the decision in this context, it becomes easier to manage. You are making a decision, based on balance, with a full understanding of the consequences. It comes down to a yes or no answer, but you can compromise with the goblin.

For example, if you stick to your strategy all week, then you will have a reward. If you give in to your desires, you have not failed completely, but you bring the possibility of doing so ever closer. You need to make the decision you want to make, not one you are manipulated into making. It is decision time, what will it be?

REINFORCE AND REACTION –

It's decision time.

Time to make your move. Before you do that though, reinforce your decision through a double check process. Reinforcement is a powerful tool to completely stop any impulse decision making.

- **Is this the right choice?**
- **Am I absolutely sure this is the right thing to do?**
- **I am fully aware of the consequences.**

So now you have to make a decision, but it is one you are making consciously having both understood and evaluated all the options. You know that whatever you decide has ramifications. You are making a decision, forgoing a few moments of pleasure in search of the long-term good. With all the facts in your possession, you will have to come up with one heck of an excuse to justify giving in to the goblin!

Are you going to give in to your cravings, and once again, be sabotaged by your inner self, or are you going to aim for a higher reward, achieving your goals and objectives? You know giving in will lead to self-loathing. Though the decision to say no is logical and a no-brainer, it is still not easy. So instead of saying 'sod-it', there are a range of tactics we can employ.

Focus more on the damage that eating this item will bring and use this as motivation to say no. Make this a decision between something that is bad for you, will do damage, and make you fat. Compare the short-term pleasure of having the item now with the long-term pleasure and benefits you will get achieving your goal. Play the long game. Focus on your primary goal and do not lose sight of that. Your primary goal, which for me was having a photo with my family in my Reiss Suit looking slim became the most important thing in my world. Tell yourself you are strong; winning this battle is an important step to winning the war.

You need to focus on an alternative way to satisfy an emotionally driven food craving. Reward yourself for not eating the chocolate (insert again as required). This can, obviously, not be a reward that has calories but an example would be to treat yourself to a book, DVD, Album, or basically anything that is a special treat. For me, it was shirts. I would buy a shirt every week when I had not had any setbacks. A lot of them now don't fit but they fulfilled their purpose.

You need to be decisive. This is important. Procrastinating, or dithering to be more precise, only increases the chances of giving in. When we dither, we create obstacles and increase the chances of capitulating. You need to adopt a ruthless decision-making streak. Focus yourself on your objectives and goals. Nothing else matters. Many leading sportsmen are notoriously selfish and have tunnel vision. Winning is everything and nothing gets in the way of that!

"Winning isn't everything, it's the only thing!"
Vince Lombardi

Rewarding good behaviour is one way to overcome giving in. The other that works well is distraction. We can divert our thinking away from this food-driven craving and focus on something else. I would take the dog for a walk when the biscuit tin seemed to have a tractor beam drawing me in. You can make a call, check your email, do some paperwork, the ironing, or anything that isn't eating and will occupy your thoughts.

You will find something that works for you, and trust me on this; it will get easier to do the right thing. In fact, as every day passes, it gets that bit easier until it becomes the norm. Whenever the goblin applies the pester pressure, implement the POWER technique. **JUST SAY NO!**

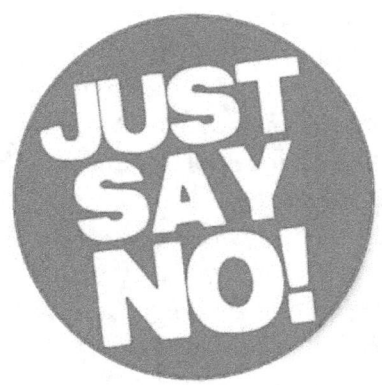

Remember the JUST SAY NO campaign? It was centred on drugs, but it is a great and memorable slogan you should adopt towards the goblin centred food cravings. It is a great slogan - Just Say No!

AN EXAMPLE OF THE POWER TECHNIQUE IN ACTION:

You are at a well-known newsagents/stationers, and you see one of their tempting offers, a giant bar of milk chocolate for only £1. It is a bargain, but chances are it will not last long either. It is full of Dairy Goodness! How did they get away with that? It is full of sugar, goodness, it isn't, but it tastes great!

There is temptation staring straight in the face, right there within easy reach. A delicious taste explosion, and the natural reaction is to have it and polish it off straight away. You have taken advantage of these offers many times before. It's almost an automatic reaction to say yes. **Now PRESS PAUSE.** You know you have to JUST SAY NO, but you are in a dilemma once again.

Reaffirm your **OBJECTIVES** and personal goals. Having this giant bar of milk chocolate is not in your long-term interests. Remember **WHY** you set your goals and how important they are to you. Your self-control mechanism will now be kicking in. Of course, you don't want to jeopardise the things you want above everything else and undo the good work you have done so far. You have to say NO.

EVALUATE the options. Short-term pleasure will be followed by self-loathing, because you will feel like a failure. Is your long-term goal more important? You bet it is. You do not give up, you do not give in, you just say NO! You have set a reward at the end of the week. So you can enjoy a guilt free reward then which will be what you want on your terms.

REINFORCE AND REACT. You are going to say NO. You will have the craving still. It won't go away just because you said no. Buy a bottle of water instead. If possible, you could have a piece of fruit. You can reward your resolve with something else, like a book or CD. After all, they sell other items, not just giant chocolate bars. When you leave the store, distract your thinking. Make a call or do something that diverts your attention from the craving. Decision made, decision reinforced, reaction is to say no, rather than the impulse to say yes.

The good news is, the more you implement the POWER technique, the more natural it becomes. This process will become second nature to you. You have taken control.

WRITE IT ALL DOWN IN YOUR FRESHPLAN JOURNAL

Keeping a Freshplan journal is a keystone habit that will significantly improve your effectiveness and give you a much greater chance of success. The simple process of logging what you consume daily has been proved to help people eat less and make healthier food choices. The Kaiser Permanente Health Research Centre in Oregon, USA, confirms the power of this technique with very clear results. In the study, nearly 1,700 overweight adults followed a healthy eating and activity programme for six months and were advised to keep daily records of what and how many calories they consumed. At the end of the study, the average weight loss was around 13lbs. There are many similar studies which reinforce these results. It has been proven the more food records people kept, the more weight they lose.

As well as journaling intake, you should also journal your successes and failures. These are two keystone habits that can transform your life.

As you encounter obstacles and learn to deal with them, write them down. As I said before, you do not need to write extensively but jot down a few notes; how you overcame the problem, and most importantly, how you felt. You will feel a great sense of achievement and control when you do the right thing. I strongly advise you to write down your thoughts EVERYDAY as you get to your target weight. Not just the good, but also the bad. Even if you write nothing else in your journal, write down whether it was a good day or a bad day!

"And bad mistakes – I've made a few. I've had my share of sand kicked in my face, But I've come through."
Queen

There is no such thing as a certainty in life, except death and taxes, and when you embark on this journey, you will make mistakes. We all do, including me, even now. However, do not view a mistake or a setback as total failure. It is just that, a setback. Mistakes and setbacks are perfectly acceptable, but giving up is not.

You are not a quitter. There is a well-known saying (or cliché depending on your point of view) that what does not kill you, only serves to make you stronger. Well, that is exactly how to view setbacks. I lost four stone and had plenty of setbacks along the way. You take casualties in war; you even sometimes lose the odd battle.

I remember once having a meltdown and polishing off a packet of Jaffa Cakes. Man, I love Jaffa Cakes. So does my partner. But coming home late, tired and fed up, I polished off the lot. I could not have felt worse the next morning. But this was a turning point for me. I never did it again, not yet anyway!

The next day, I spoke to my partner about it, and she said when you have such a setback, you need to *'get on it like a car bonnet'* the next day and learn from it. You cannot change the past, but you can influence the future.

"What is done is done. Forget the past and focus on the future."
Carl Harris

When you were a baby, learning to walk, you fell over again and again, yet you got up and tried again. Eventually, you stopped falling over and started to walk then you got better at walking and eventually, you stopped falling over all together. If only we were as resilient as adults, nothing would stop us. As adults, we are meant to be wiser and stronger, yet we give up much more easily than we did as a child. If you have a setback, learn from it. All humans make mistakes. The key is to make less from now going forward. Learning from these mistakes is what will ensure we eventually reach our goals. The only true failure is giving up altogether!

By journaling the things you did right and what you feel you should have done when things went wrong, you will create a ready-made set of 'what if' plans. Having an arsenal to deal with potential pitfalls puts you in a strong position. It is important to not merely write in your journal, but also to review it regularly. When you plan for situations that can challenge your resolve, you reduce the risk of giving in.

Consequently, it is better to proactively prevent cravings happening in the first place, instead of having to deal with them. When you acknowledge your darker emotions, they have less power over you. The pen is mighty. It is your secret weapon. Do not underestimate the effect your journal will have in helping you make big changes.

Treat a setback as an opportunity. Setbacks can be beneficial in the long run if they are treated as successful learning experiences. If you read the biographies of successful people in business, politics or sport, you will hear one theme repeated over and over, which is people learn more from failure than they do from success. If you have a setback, analyse why it happened, write down what happened in your journal and resolve it will not happen again with the same set of circumstances. By doing this, you will be ready and can deploy your defences if the situation arises in future. Your mantra from now on with the Freshplan is very simple, "I will not fail."

'Celebrate it when it is successful; reward it when it is successful; and learn from failure by not making the same mistakes twice.'
Justin King

You should also celebrate your successes. Do not spend all your time dwelling on failures. Be sure to rejoice in your achievements. If you spend all your time examining failure, you will develop a negative Mindset. You need to have a positive frame of mind, expect to succeed and make sure you are always in control. The more you can enjoy the process, the more effective you will be. Life is meant to be fun after all.

No one has ever achieved their dreams by giving up, because it turned out to be harder than they thought it was going to be. My grandfather told me many years ago:

"Life is easy when you live it the hard way"
John Hacking

Your past may define you, but it doesn't control your future. Learn from the mistakes made in the past and use them to shape a better future. It is easy to stick with easy. Instant gratification is easy, saying sod-it is easy, and letting the goblin dictate what you eat is easy. Sticking with easy will not achieve your goals. Easy is easy, but look what easy has done for you so far!

Avoiding repeating the same mistakes you made in the past and making a change is what you need to do. One of the best quotes of all time comes from Albert Einstein:

"Insanity is doing the same thing over and over expecting different results."

This is the best reason I know to adopt a fresh approach. For years, I tried and failed to lose weight. I expected different results every time, but never achieved anything but more failure. That is why I devised Freshplan. Everything else failed. If this is the same for you, then rather than be despondent, you should feel positive about the fact you have not given up. Never give up. You never fail until you have given up altogether.

Remember this:

"Winners Never Quit and Quitters Never Win."

INTRODUCING 'SOD-IT' SATURDAYS

Celebrating successes, for example having a good week and losing weight, is important. This is a balancing act, but rewards are extremely important. You need a bit of sweet with the sour, quite literally, in this case.

You must not go overboard. I recommend you escalate your rewards as you achieve more weight loss. What I did was have a 'Sod-it Saturday'. When I started, I would work towards Saturday night. If I had a good week with no setbacks and lost weight, I allowed myself a treat. At first, this was a Mars Bar or bag of crisps. As the weeks passed and my weight came off, I increased the level of rewards. Now I am at my target weight. If I maintain it for the week I have Saturday as a full cheat day because I have earned it and it gives me something to work towards. It doesn't have to be Saturday, of course, but once a week you should toast your success.

I would stress that the level of reward you have must be reasonable. There is no point in going all out on sod-it Saturday in the early stages of your Freshplan, as you will undo all the work you have done. Make your rewards exciting but reasonable.

DELAYED GRATIFICATION

One craving counter measure you can employ is to delay gratification until sod-it Saturday. Your goblin is seeking instant gratification. By delaying gratification until sod-it Saturday, you reach a compromise. For example, if you have a craving for Jaffa Cakes, you can write in your journal at the top of Saturday's page that your reward is two Jaffa Cakes. This gives you an incentive to work towards a reward you really want. This works extremely well.

Rewards are extremely important. Break down your progression into one week at a time. Work towards achieving your reward at the end of your week.

To achieve success, we need to make our human brain the default thinking machine, instead of letting our emotions and greedy goblin call the shots. Remember, the first thoughts that rush into your head craving food come from that goblin living in your chimp brain. Your journal is so important. All you need is to spend just 10 minutes at the end of each day to reflect on your thoughts and actions from the day.

Categorize them into goblin and human responses. This will help you recognize where you went right, as well as wrong. You must understand the goblin and the chimp brain only make suggestions and it's your human brain that carries out the actions. This means you have, as you always have, control of what you do. Now you have the POWER to stop making snap, emotionally driven decisions and make sensible, rational choices.

Your goblin can not be changed, silenced, or killed. You are stuck with it as long as you are alive. And so is the goblin demanding food. It will always be there, waiting to take control. So managing it is the best you can do, but in managing it, you can reason with it using your human brain, the more you manage it, the easier it becomes, and the greater your control will be.

In the end, you have a choice whether to think as a goblin or as a human. This is the key to success. If you conquer this, then success will be easy. Rome was not built in a day (sorry another cliché), so it will take time, but do not stop trying. Keep your objectives in sight at all times, implement the POWER process, and never doubt that success will happen. If you do have a setback along the way, it is not the end. Remember this:

"The only way you can truly fail with the Freshplan is to quit."

THE FRESHPLAN 10 GOLDEN RULES:

1. Start your Freshplan Journal.
2. Write down your starting stats (weight and measurements etc.)
3. Define your objectives (the numbers you want to achieve).
4. Set out your personal goals (keep it short and sweet).

5. Use the **POWER** Process when you have food cravings. Press **PAUSE**, restate your **OBJECTIVES**, ask yourself **WHY?** Then **EVALUATE** all the options before you **REACT** and make a conscious decision. Remember **JUST SAY NO!**
6. Spend 10 minutes every day to update your journal with good and bad events and any setbacks.
7. Setbacks - no problem, learn from them, write down what you will do next time if the same situation arises. Use them as a positive learning experience.
8. Review your journal once a week.
9. Introduce a reward system at the end of your week. Increase the reward as time goes by and your weight loss increases.
10. A setback is not failure, the only failure is giving up!

PREPARE YOUR BATTLE PLAN FOR THE DAY AHEAD

Foresight is better than hindsight. Failing to prepare is preparing to fail, which is yet another cliché, but another which is spot on. The best way to prevent being ambushed by your goblin is to be ready. Take your Freshplan one day at a time. Each day is a battle. Keep winning battles, and you will soon win the war. If you focus on today, making sure it is a good day, you are another step closer to achieving your objectives and goals.

I have found that focusing on one day at a time is the easiest way to maintain motivation and stay on plan. Though no two days are the same, you have a fairly good idea of what lies ahead in the morning. Use the following guide to prepare for the potential problems you may face.

1. **Refocus.** Recite or read your objectives and goals every morning. This will reaffirm what is important to you and every day brings you a step closer to achieving them. Do this every morning.
2. **Review the success you have had to date**. This will reaffirm what you will be putting in jeopardy if you give into temptation.
3. **Look forward to the day ahead** and identify any obvious hazards. For example, if you are meeting a friend for coffee, don't be tempted to have a cake but you know you will be. You know what you need to eat, set it out, and stick to what is on your diet plan.
4. **Set Goals for the day.** Not just the goal of staying on your diet plan, but you can set other goals. If your mind is occupied then its focus will be elsewhere other than food cravings.
5. **Be ready!** You know you can be called upon at any time to fend off cravings at any time. You also have a series of what if scenarios in place and the tools to overcome any obstacle you encounter.

You may start every day with good intentions, but if your track record has been one of repeated failure where your weight is concerned, organisation will focus your thought process. By doing this every morning you will make the right choices. Another cliché is you need to sing from the diet's hymn sheet, so being aware of it means you know the words, and you will not mess up.

There is also a scientific principle behind advance planning. When you are planning, you are in a cold state. The cravings and temptations are not clouding your judgement and you can think clearly. This is known as 'resistant bias.' This is perfectly illustrated when people do their supermarket shopping online and they spend less than when they do it in store. They fall prey to the temptation before their eyes with the sights, sounds and smells in the shops, which have been scientifically optimised for that very purpose.

Think of the morning after. Do you want to wake up tomorrow knowing you have failed? Of course not, and you know all you have to do to stop that from happening is say no when the goblin comes calling.

You will see the benefit of planning your day in advance, not just with your weight loss and management, but in other parts of your life too. For the time you take in doing this, the reward is huge. Give it a try.

Chapter 11
Freshplan keystone weight loss tactics

Managing your decision making process is the key to weight loss success. However, to achieve the best results, I have created the Freshplan Weight Loss toolkit to make the weight loss and weight management process easier. Again, these techniques and tools can be used in conjunction with any diet you follow.

Part two of this book will detail the Freshplan Diet. I would urge you to follow this diet but it is the ability to stick to your chosen diet that is the most important aspect. These tricks, tools and techniques can be universally adopted. Once again, they are all the subject of both research and implementation and will help you achieve your goals quicker. Work smarter, not harder!

One thing I have found in my forty five years on Earth is most people over-complicate life and get bogged down in the detail. My view is to focus on the big issues and the minutia will fall into place. Working 'Smarter Not Harder' will serve you well in life, more so when it comes to losing weight.

I spoke earlier about MARGINAL GAINS, the concept of making small changes that add up to big changes and better results. These are what I would term as weight loss marginal gains. They take little effort to implement but deliver significant results.

One thing I will stress, right now, is your nutritional habits will have a far greater impact on your weight loss efforts than any other component. Sticking to your diet plan is what will lose weight. There is no short cut. No miracle pill will work. Even with gastric surgery, all that does is make you incapable of taking in more calories than you need. It is the ultimate white flag of defeat.

Losing weight, when you break it down, is actually a very straightforward process. As we know, it is not easy for us to do but the process of shedding excess weight is a simple one. Consume less energy than you burn on a daily basis. Without controlling your food intake, you will not lose weight. You can lose weight through dieting alone. You will not lose weight purely through exercise if you eat and drink to excess. If you hate any form of exercise, that is good news. That is not to say there is no point in exercising because the more you move, the more calories you burn, and of course, it is good for your health.

I have used the phrase KEYSTONE HABITS several times. Your life is probably already full of keystone habits, many of which have a detrimental effect on your health and weight. Keystone habits are habits and behaviours which automatically lead to changes in other behaviours, creating a chain of unconscious level events. The Freshplan recommends implementing a series of beneficial keystone habits for maximum benefit. These are very easy to adopt.

Keystone habits are where to focus, rather than wasting your time with ineffective, less important things. Research suggests it takes 21 uses to memorize something and about a month of doing something every day to turn it into a habit. Get this right, and magic will happen before your eyes.

These are the Freshplan Keystone Habits to focus on:

DRINK WATER - VITALLY IMPORTANT TO YOUR SUCCESS

I am not telling you anything you don't know but our bodies are up to 70% water. This figure can vary quite wildly, depending on what you read, but once again, no point in getting bogged down in that. It is safe to say a human contains more water than anything else put together. So it is no surprise that we need to drink plenty of water.

The more coffee, alcohol and soft drinks you consume, the more water you need to drink. The Freshplan advocates, during the initial phase of reaching your target weight, you drink water and all other drinks are rationed and used only as rewards.

The list of benefits that drinking water brings is huge. We can live without food for much longer than you can without water. Your energy levels depend on you drinking sufficient water. Water flushes the toxins from your body. Without enough water, your thought process is impaired. You will, therefore, be more vulnerable to your goblin if you are not thinking as sharply as usual.

Drink more water. Do this from now on for the rest of your life. Even if you abandon everything in this book, never stop drinking water. It keeps you hydrated without calories. You may not be aware of this; I certainly was surprised, but your body sometimes misinterprets thirst as hunger, so drinking water will help you eat less. Keep yourself hydrated. Always. When you're dehydrated, your brain pumps out more vasopressin, a hormone that tells your liver to produce glucose. A sugar fuelled diet with insufficient water is the perfect recipe for diabetes.

These are just some of the benefits of drinking water:

- Drink a large glass of water, at least, preferably two, first thing every morning.
- When you feel hungry, try drinking water first; the hunger may have been thirst.
- Before every meal, drink two glasses of ice cold water. This will fill you up and stop overeating. Drinking ice-cold water has been proven to burn calories!
- Studies have shown that people who drink two glasses of water before eating a meal consume fewer calories and can lose half-a-stone in weight due to this alone.
- Sip water with your meal and you will fill faster.
- Water boosts your metabolism, stimulates your brain function and boosts your immune system, helps your blood sugar levels, cholesterol, you name it, water helps. Water is the most beneficial single thing your body takes in.

Until you hit your target weight, you should drink only the following:

- Water, drink ice-cold water all day long. Keep yourself hydrated, around five pints a day.
- Only one coffee a day, skimmed milk
- No alcohol of any kind at all. We will discuss later

EAT SLOWER, CHEW YOUR FOOD AND GO JAPANESE

Research shows eating more slowly helps people eat less, perhaps, because it allows our brain time to communicate when we are full and allows extra time for the body to digest food. Researchers from Texas Christian University explored the relationship between eating speed and calorie intake by looking at how eating speed affects calories consumed during a meal. The study found eating slowly and having smaller bites makes us feel less hungry an hour afterwards than if we wolf down food. People who ate slowly also drank more, which helped them feel fuller for longer. Taking smaller bites helps us digest food more effectively. It is a Keystone Habit you need to consciously change. A small change with big benefits.

Confucianism (an old Chinese proverb) teaches HARA HACHI BU, which is eating until 80% full. Not overeating may be easier advice to follow, as how do you know when you reach 80%? Nature, sadly, has not given us a dial like you would find in a car. The proverb says:

"Eight parts of a full stomach sustain the man; the other two sustain the doctor."

By eating slower and chewing more, you will be more in tune with your body. Try to not eat until you are full, and certainly, when you feel you are full, STOP EATING.

BUY SMALLER PLATES AND YOU ARE NOT MAGNUS MAGNUSSON

This may sound like really obvious advice but just because you have started it doesn't mean you have to finish. Of course, Magnus Magnusson was the former host of TV's 'Mastermind' and had the catchphrase, "I've started so I'll finish." That does not apply to eating and this is a great example of a keystone habit that is doing us harm.

As children we are conditioned to finish our plate. Indeed, I was always told I had to finish my meal or face the consequences. This was done with good intentions, of course, but a parent wanting to ensure their child is well-nourished paradoxically is training them to overeat as second nature. As we repeatedly finish the portion we are given, so it becomes second nature and we grow up subconsciously programmed to always finish what is before us. You do not need to!

One way to counteract this is to buy smaller plates. You will probably not have noticed this but I was told by someone in the pottery trade that the average size of a main course plate is now 50% bigger than 25 years ago. So get smaller plates. If you do find yourself unable to leave anything on your plate, having a smaller portion to begin with has served a beneficial purpose.

Become aware of when you are full. Research has shown that eating as a secondary activity leads to overeating. This means if you eat watching TV, for example, you are more likely to eat more food than if you sat down at the table and focused solely on eating. They key is to take all food choices and eating related activities out of your subconscious and into your conscious thought process.

After you repeat these processes, your brain will rewrite its automatic processes and bad habits will be replaced with good habits.

10K EVERYDAY

Do not panic. I am not suggesting you run ten kilometres every day! I am referring to the number of steps you take every day. If you have a smart phone, you can download a free pedometer app that will measure your daily steps. You can buy pedometers for only a few pounds. You might be surprised how little you actually move in the course of a day.

Walking is essential, obviously, but if you get tired walking any sort of distance then consider this a red flag. Of course, if you have a genuine medical reason for doing so then disregard that, but if the only reason is you are overweight and unfit, this needs addressing. Make it a priority to walk at least ten thousand steps every day. By the way, the day that shows 6,000 steps in the photo, I left my phone at home, so the data is incomplete, honest!

The average person's stride length is approximately 2.5 feet long. That means it takes just over 2,000 steps to walk one mile and 10,000 steps is close to five miles. With modern life and a sedentary job, people now walk as little as 1,000 to 3,000 steps a day. This is nowhere near enough. For the first seven days simply measure the steps you take, living life normally. You will be surprised. Walking more will have immediate benefits. Walking can help you build stamina, burn excess calories and give you a healthier heart.

This is a keystone habit. Make it a golden rule to walk 10,000 steps every day. Taking a dog for a walk is a great way of achieving this. Walk your dog further; it will appreciate it. If you don't have a dog, there is no reason not to go for a walk. Replace short car journeys with a walk and take the stairs instead of a lift.

Clocking up 10k steps everyday will have enormous benefits. You will feel fitter, healthier and happier. You will burn up to 400 extra calories a day. Your brain will also start to release endorphins. These are not reserved for muscle clad gym bunnies; you can get the benefits of them too. Endorphins trigger a positive feeling in the body, similar to that of morphine. If you enjoy it, you will want to do it again. Walking 10k steps a day is not at all arduous and for the effort involved, you get hugely rewarded.

SLEEP - ALWAYS GET A GOOD 7 HOURS OF SLEEP

This is a keystone habit, which literally involves doing absolutely nothing at all! Getting at least seven hours a night of sleep will have huge benefits in all aspects of life. The better your sleep pattern, the lower your stress levels will be.

People who aren't getting enough sleep and are under stress may have more difficulty sticking to a weight loss programme. However, this association does not mean that poor sleep causes obesity, or healthy sleep patterns are a means of achieving weight loss. If you think about this logically, the more alert you are, the stronger your thinking will be. When you are not as alert, your defences are lowered and the goblin will strike. Sleep is so important.

If you have had trouble sleeping in the past, the chances are your diet has been a huge contributor. Eating a healthy diet will help sleep. Sleeping well will help your food choices. They are both keystone habits, directly influencing one another. There is a plethora of research about the effects of sleep but you do not need to get bogged down in all that. I think it is safe to say no one will challenge the notion that sleep is good for you. Make sure you get seven hours sleep a night. Do not sleep more than eight hours a night; too much sleep is not good for you either.

When you go to bed, you go to bed to sleep. Do not do anything else in bed, other than sleep or have sex. No reading, no TV, absolutely no phone, tablet or laptop. The light that is emitted from these stimulate your brain and can prevent sleep or cause poor quality sleep.

If you suffer from insomnia and are unable to cure it, see a doctor, but do not, I repeat do not, take sleeping pills. You will see a benefit in the short-term but in the long-term you will have more problems. There will be an answer to your problem but sleeping pills is not the answer.

Many people who have sleep issues have a magnesium deficiency. Try taking some magnesium supplements for a quick fix. You may be surprised how a big problem is so easily solved.

TAKE A DAILY PROBIOTIC AND EAT MORE GARLIC

I do not like supplements and vitamins etc because if you follow a healthy, balanced and nutritious diet, you do not need them. There are two I take every day without fail. Probiotic and garlic. Probiotics are also known as good or friendly bacteria.

Taking a probiotic every day is one of the best things you can do. Gut health is rapidly growing in importance in the medical world. Giulia Enders book, *The Inside Story of The Gut* is a fascinating read. She argues that the influence of the gut on our health and wellbeing is one of the new lines of research in modern medicine!

Enders states: "It is now generally accepted in scientific circles that people with certain digestive problems often suffer from nervous disorders of the gut. Their gut then sends signals to the part of the brain that processes negative feelings, although they have done nothing bad." It may sound clichéd but if you look after the gut, it will look after you.

Unhealthy gut flora can negatively impact your mental health, potentially leading to issues like anxiety, depression, attention deficit and an all-round negative outlook. A recent study has proven that regularly consuming beneficial bacteria will improve your brain function.

Just as you have neurons in your brain, you also have neurons in your gut, including neurons that produce neurotransmitters like serotonin, which is also found in your brain and is a mood enhancer. Limiting sugar, eating traditionally fermented foods and taking a probiotic supplement are among the best ways to optimize your gut flora and, subsequently, support your brain health and normalise your mood.

One of the many negative side effects created by a manufactured food diet is the good bacteria our gut needs to work effectively is not being consumed in sufficient volume. Sweet cravings may be caused by an imbalance in the gut microflora (gut bacteria). Taking garlic every day can kill harmful bacteria and yeast that grow in your gut. Much is spoken about yeast imbalances but you need do no more than take probiotic and garlic. Again, we have no need to get bogged down in the detail.

Probiotics will help stop sugar cravings and like all good keystone habits, they have knock on positive effects too. It will improve your immune system and you will get fewer colds, if any next winter. You will see improvements in your skin and hair appearance (if you have any), and overall, your general wellbeing will be better. There are different types of probiotics. Again, I do not get bogged down in the detail; I simply alternate the brands I buy. Remember, a better diet will also improve your gut bacteria, particularly from fresh vegetable consumption.

Do not buy probiotic drinks from the supermarket. You are better with a probiotic tablet from a health food shop. As you have probably already realised, you cannot trust manufactured products. I will place a bet with you now. If you know anyone who says they suffer from IBS (irritable bowel syndrome), tell them to take a probiotic every day for a month and at the end of it, they will be delighted with the result. Most IBS is a result of the lack of good bacteria in the gut. As Giulia Enders, a Doctor, points out, most doctors learn very little about this during their training.

You can take it from me that the benefits of a daily probiotic are immense, not only for you but for those you live with! Garlic is also extremely good for you in other ways, particularly your heart. The World Health Organisation now recommends you consume a clove of garlic every day. It has so many health benefits but of course it smells. I personally take garlic via a capsule because it is tasteless and odourless. This is for the love of my friends and family primarily because there is no improving on anything that is fresh and natural but sometimes compromises have to be made.

Probiotics and garlic every day is a small change that has big beneficial effects. Make this mandatory from now on and you will notice the benefits within a very short space of time.

TRICKS TO SPEED UP YOUR METABOLISM

Metabolism is a huge topic, but in short, this is the rate at which your body burns energy. There are some subtle ways in which you can speed up your metabolism. The best way is to do some weight training twice a week but for those who neither have the time nor the inclination to do this, these are small changes that can impact on your metabolism:

- Drink water first thing in a morning
- Have a cold shower, or finish your shower on cold, this kick starts your metabolism.
- Walk before you have breakfast in a morning, ideally a jog.
- Turn the central heating down a couple of degrees.
- Eat spicy food, e.g. chillies, twice a week. Chillies are potent metabolism-boosters. Just one chilli can speed up your metabolism by as much as 25% within three hours.
- Avoid Alcohol. We will cover alcohol in detail shortly but it will slow down your metabolism, dramatically.
- Eat good quality, fresh fruit and vegetables every day. The better the quality of food you eat, the faster your body can metabolise it.

There may be other tricks you can add to the list, but remember, there is a danger of overload. Treat this as a mental bandwidth issue. There is only so much capacity. The more selective and focused you are, the more successful you will be.

Chapter 12
Freshplan self-help

I wanted to conclude this section with some words of wisdom and personal advice. I strongly believe the difference between success and failure has more to do with your Mindset than anything else. I have read countless self-help books, ranging from the ridiculous to the brilliant. There is so much more reading you can do. The more you understand about how your mind works the better. The key to success is to believe you will always succeed, never contemplate failure and never give it a moment's thought; from now on failure does not exist.

On the journey you are starting, you have a route map in place. You know where you are going and indeed how to get there; however, there will be bumps and obstacles along that road which you know will be there but you don't know exactly what, where and when these will be. But we have put plans in place to deal with them.

The Freshplan is proactive, rather than reactive. You have the tools to overcome any obstacle you may face along the way. By having the right Mindset in place with the tools to deal with all eventualities, you have the recipe for success.

The key is to stay motivated. When the motivation level starts to dip, it is worth reviewing your journal and your results. Keeping focus will lead to success.

"Just because we know the best way forward doesn't mean we'll actually take it."
Paul McGee (SUMO)

SUMO (by Paul McGee) is a great book to read. It puts things into perspective and you will get plenty out of it. *SUMO* points out that when the event or the problem is happening to someone else, it's easier for you to take a more objective perspective. The less emotionally involved you are, the easier it is to engage your rational brain than when the issue affects you directly. That is a great approach to take. I think back to the conversation I had with my partner after a late night meltdown, "What would she say?"

We almost always know what the common sense approach is, but we do not always take it. Advising yourself in the third person is a technique I adopted for myself. Try it, it really works. I recently thanked my partner for her advice on an issue; she thought she was losing the plot because it was advice I had given myself from her in the third person. It sounds crazy but it is a technique that works time after time.

'What would (insert name as required) say?'

I have found the 'What would Sharon say' approach works on my chimp brain as a whole not just the goblin in that part of the brain. It doesn't like being ganged-up on, and by adopting this technique I can silence it very easily. It is a great Mindset tactic to bring into play. The key for me is the excuses I would previously have offered up for giving in and saying sod-it are headed off at the pass and invalidated, leaving nowhere to go but to make the right decision and stay strong. It works for me and has worked for others. Give it a try.

THE DISCIPLINED ME APPROACH

I can up with a twist on my 'What Would Sharon Say' approach. He doesn't listen to anyone, so he now takes the advice of the 'me he wants to be'. We agreed he has been Despicable Me for far too long, so now he wants to become a new and improved *'Disciplined Me'*.

This could be an approach that works for you. Construct, in your mind, the person you want to be, one who looks like you want to look, having achieved your goals. There is no point in doing this and transforming yourself into Brad Pitt or Angelina Jolie because that isn't going to happen.

The 'Disciplined Me' will be strong, decisive and wise and, by definition, is the person you aspire to be. If you start to think like and act like the disciplined, strategic thinking winner you aspire to be, you will eventually transform into that person. By following this approach, my friend says every day he becomes more like the ideal version of himself he aspires to be. Give it a try!

Just for clarity here, I am not advocating you literally start talking to yourself out loud, this is a thought process. I do not want you to start looking like you have gone insane. That said, I recently started reading *'The Good Psychopath's Guide'* by Kevin Dutton and Andy McNab. They are fascinating to read and, without any doubt, decision making would be so much easier if we were psychopaths. No conflict there. We wouldn't have to worry about emotional responses and could utilise our human brain all the time.

I advocate reading self-help books about your thought processes because the more you learn, the more skilled you become. But be selective. Dutton and McNab offer an excellent mix of academic and practical application. In a review of their book it said, "Our Good Psychopath Manifesto will transform you from someone who pussyfoots about on the left to a dynamic, go-getting achiever who maxes out on the right." I simply had to read it. But there is a serious point to this.

The one person who will, ultimately, determine whether you succeed or fail is just you, no one else. You really have it within you not only to fulfil your personal objectives and goals, but to take that one step forward and inspire and mentor others to do the same in future. Taking advice, learning and being willing to accept and embrace change will serve you well. Stop dithering and start doing.

Just as failure is contagious, success is infectious, and people will want to share whatever magic they perceive has happened to you. You will be so different that people will notice, both your physical and character changes. I met someone who I had not seen for a couple of years at York races recently. He literally walked past me and smiled until I said hello. He was stunned. He apologised, saying he was not being rude but he genuinely didn't recognise me. He said I looked 10 years younger, so different and he wanted to follow my lead. These are great reactions, which will happen to you too!

Though we are all unique, all humans share several traits, one of which is fragility. You will make mistakes. We all do; I certainly do even now. When you do make a mistake, learn from it and move on. That is why I can identify with the SUMO principle, Shut Up and Move On. Every day is a clean piece of paper in your Freshplan Journal to be filled with success. The future hasn't happened yet. You can influence your future, be the driver, or you can sit back and let it happen.

If you opt for the latter, there is no doubt you will end up somewhere you don't want to be. Getting your Mindset right is the key that will give you the power over your future. When you are in control, you dictate the direction of travel.

Once you are able to constantly focus your mind and take charge of subconscious actions by thinking consciously and focusing on the outcome you want, you will easily make it happen. This never fails, which means you now have total control over your life. If you allow your chimp brain to take over, and the goblin to run riot, you run the risk of sabotaging all the good work you have done. Focus is, therefore, the key. Remember to press PAUSE and use the POWER technique before you make any decision.

"Taking personal responsibility frees you from the trap of blaming, complaining, and resenting."
Paul McGee (SUMO)

Excuses are not valid anymore because you have the tools to resist temptation. You are the master of your own destiny, so take full responsibility. You can do it, and you will do it!

THE WWW OF WHAT YOU EAT

Earlier, I spoke about breaking down your journey into one day at a time. If you boil it down to the lowest common denominator, you will realise this is won one mouthful at a time. You accept that you have control of what you put in your mouth, you have a series of thought processes to go through, POWER, STOP LOOK AND LISTEN and JUST SAY NO, but there is another layer you may choose to add.

I have devised a simple formula. Although this will never trouble the Nobel Panel, it is very effective:

W+W+W = YES

When you eat or drink, or anything for that matter, must meet a simple criteria, dictated by your weight loss objectives. Each W relates to three elements:

- **WHAT?** - is what you are about to eat part of your diet plan, is it good for you, or is it an authorised reward? Is it in the right quantity, i.e. not over your allocation?

- **WHY?** - If the answer to the above is yes, then this is a moot point, but do you have a valid reason or are you eating as a result of cravings or emotional triggers?

- **WHEN?** – Are you eating at the right time, at meal times, for example? You shouldn't eat after 7pm, only drink, so are you breaking your culinary curfew?

Only if you get three x YES are you allowed to eat or drink the item in question. As I said, not at all scientific but it makes you consciously authorise everything that passes your lips. Having gone through all these processes you really should find it impossible to break your diet.

DON'T EAT AFTER 7PM

One of the best weight loss tips, which is easy to implement, is to impose a 7pm curfew on food consumption. Put a blanket ban on any form of food, or drink for that matter, except water of course, after 7pm. Now if you work shifts, clearly this doesn't apply but for the vast majority of us who keep regular hours, this is a habit you should adopt for life.

It is common sense really. Your daily meals have finished, your calorie consumption for the day has been taken aboard but, more importantly, your calorie burning is also complete for the day.

Any food you take on after 7pm is excess food, outside of your meal plan and likely to be some form of treat. It is unnecessary, that is for sure. If you are watching TV, eating can become secondary, and a couple of crisps out of a bag can escalate subconsciously until the whole bag is gone.

This curfew includes alcohol and coffee. Both are neuro-stimulants and without them before sleep, you will find you have a much better sleep. Just have water. You will find you wake with much more energy and a clearer head.

Scientifically, your body has no idea what time it is. There is no physiological reason why eating after 7pm is any different than eating before, but in studies where this was implemented, participants lost weight as a rule. The reason though was simple. They consumed fewer calories daily than they otherwise would. Every time!

Looking at this through the common sense filter, which is always the best way, it makes perfect sense that cutting out nothing more than top-up calories is bound to have an effect. Also by imposing this curfew, a strong defence is always in place, a defence against sod-it mode.

When you relax in the evening, you are more likely to have cravings because your mind is less occupied than throughout the day. Snacking in front of the TV is probably a bad habit you have picked up over the years; I know it has been for me.

It is easier to not have anything than to have just one. If not eating after 7pm becomes a golden rule and way of life, you will feel the benefit. I promise you.

Most diets are broken after 7pm and the calories consumed at night are excess ones and low quality. By executive order, a 7pm curfew applies. It works, I promise you!

FRESHPLAN INNERCIRCLE MANAGEMENT

The people you surround yourself with can be critical to your resolve and, ultimately, your success. The core is your home life, your immediate family, those you love and those who love you. Your family will help you and, by definition, you can count on their support.

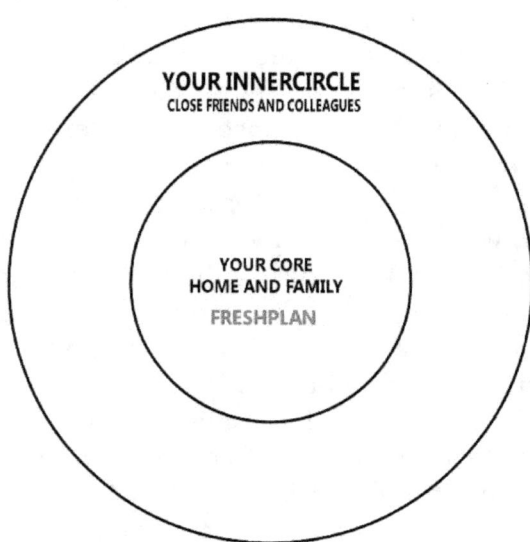

Your inner circle is made up of your close friends and colleagues, who you bring in from the outside world and bring them closer to you. These people can play a huge part in your success or otherwise.

You need to surround yourself with people who will energise you with positive support and encouragement. The opposite of energisers are sappers or drainers and these people can have a negative effect and jeopardise your chances of success.

If you have a friend who also wants to lose weight then working as a team will keep you both motivated and accountable. You will also benefit from being able to talk things through with each other, keep each other going and provide help when the going gets tough.

> *'Tough times don't last. Tough people do.'*
> Floyd Mayweather

It has been proven that by involving or associating with positive people, those who energise, will enhance your chances of success and minimise the chances of failure. If you have a family member (you can choose your friends) or friend/colleague that is negative, my advice is not to share what you are doing with them. Nowadays, people hide behind the term banter, when it really is personal and undermining. So do not allow them the opportunity to do it. What they don't know about they can't act upon.

Your chimp brain thrives on praise and complements and, as humans, we seek the approval of those we respect and admire. Therefore, having the right people aboard as you embark on this life-changing journey is hugely important. The key difference is that a positive energising person will give you the motivation to keep going and will genuinely be pleased for you.

Many people are very insecure and their insecurity manifests itself in many negative forms. These include jealousy and envy. There are plenty of people who will either openly, or secretly, take great pleasure in seeing you fail. Having these people in your inner circle is a bad move. My advice is lock them out.

I must explain what that means before you go falling out with long-term friends. You can have different inner circles for different areas of your life. They can be event or activity driven. You will have professional, social, and family inner circles. They sometimes overlap, but with regards to your weight loss and weight management, you can create an inner circle with a blank piece of paper. You may want to tell everyone you know, so you have pressure to achieve results. Most people do not thrive under such pressure, as I said we are all different. Do what is right for you but you must not involve negative people. They are dangerous and will eventually wear you down.

In this modern age of social media, you may decide to go public and go into detail on social media, letting the world know. The choice is yours but let me address a few potential problems you may face. First, are Facebook friends, real friends? I am staggered by the people I know who have huge numbers of Facebook friends but when broken down, a big percentage of those are people they have never met and only know through Facebook. At least Facebook has privacy controls and you can manage who you interact with.

Twitter is open to the world and now we live in an online world which has changed the human personality. First, everyone is now an expert on absolutely anything. You can't reason with an idiot so my view is, why bother? There is a danger of getting advice overload. If you have a plan, stick to it.

You are looking for support from your inner circle not weight loss tips and consultation.

I am staggered by the number of armchair experts, usually overweight, who offer me weight loss advice. I believe you never stop learning but unless someone has put something into practice and can back up the advice, in my view, it has no merit.

Second, people now display what I call Twitter Bravery. In normal social situations, people wouldn't say many of the things they do online to each other. These keyboard warriors are not limited by their internal social mechanisms. If you take men talking to women online, many of these Twitter artists would not dare approach a woman, never mind say some of the stuff they are happy to say online.

Similarly, people become much more aggressive online. Curtis Woodhouse, a footballer turned boxer, famously tracked down someone who was being abusive to him, posting a picture of the street sign where he lived. Quickly backtracking, the guy tweeted: 'I am sorry it's getting a bit out of hand. I am in the wrong. I accept that.' Woodhouse eventually went home and later, jokingly, tweeted: 'Just found out you can block people. Could have let me know earlier. I could have saved 20 quid in petrol.'

This illustrates perfectly the Twitter bravery in action. The choice is yours and joining a community of likeminded people, with the same objectives may be better for you online, rather than potentially involving the lunatic fringe lurking online. I strongly suggest limiting the number of people you involve to the select few you invite into your inner circle.

There will be bumps in the road along the way when you are more susceptible to succumbing to temptation. Watch out for diet saboteurs. They usually are found in social situations and peer pressure.

An example is when you are with friends, having a drink. You are sticking to sparkling water but your friends start encouraging you to have a drink. They are doing the goblin's bidding; 'One won't hurt', 'You lost weight so you've earned it', they will come thick and fast. Diet Saboteurs do not like change. They may not be doing it deliberately. It might be a case that they simply miss the old you.

This is where you need the right person to be on board, in the light of just one dissenting voice the group pressure is likely to abate. You need to remain resolute.

KINDNESS, LAUGHTER AND GRATITUDE CAN HELP TOO

Happiness is good for the soul. It makes you feel better, it makes you feel positive and that has a knock-on effect in all aspects of your life. Life is short, so enjoy it. Happiness though is a key determinant of how successful you are in both your personal and professional life. There are more reasons to be happy than to be miserable, that's for sure.

Happiness doesn't just come from being successful; it leads to success. The effects of a happy Mindset are huge. By being happy you will be a more sociable person, you will be more positive in your outlook and you will be more motivated to strive towards the goals you have defined. So as all really fat people claim to be happy, they have an advantage for losing the weight!

Research is conclusive. Happiness is positive for the human body. Happier people have stronger immune systems than miserable ones! I know what you are thinking now. I can't just magically become happy. That is a very fair point.

Happiness is not financial; the best route to happiness has to do with some very simple things. Doing a favour for someone, opening doors for people, allowing people to pass first are small acts of kindness. Smile at people, say hello to strangers, just do things a nice person would do. Very quickly, your body kicks in to a happy mode. From this happy mode, your whole outlook, motivation and Mindset become positively charged. You will feel great as your brain releases hormones that give you a natural good feeling.

You have the power to determine 50% of your happiness, with the other 50% being genetically determined. Of the remaining half, only 10% is governed by environmental factors, so you are, through your behaviour, able to influence how you act and interact with the people around you. We can get bogged down in the minefield of advice that is available about being happy, but in simple terms, if you act nice and do nice things, happiness follows. We all strive to be smiley, happy people, so what's the harm in being one?

CHOOSING THE RIGHT DIET PLAN

You might think it is ridiculous to say, but the actual diet strategy you adopt is almost secondary. The Freshplan Diet, in section 2 of this book, is very effective, easy and enjoyable. The reality is the majority of diets will get you to where you want to be if you stick to them. As we have discussed in detail, sticking to diets is the reason most people fail.

There are some good ones, but there are some ludicrous ones out there. Mainstream diets, like Slimming World and Weight Watchers, are perfectly adequate diet plans as long as you stay on plan. You must follow a nutritionally balanced diet. I would strongly advise you do not do anything extreme. The no carb diet, fasting diets and the Dukan Diet, in my view, should be avoided. You do not need to put yourself through it.

According to the British Dietetic Association (BDA), the top diets to avoid are as follows:

The Dukan diet: This restrictive, complicated diet includes phases of eating only protein and avoiding a number of foods. The BDA says, 'There is absolutely no solid science behind this at all' and cutting out food groups is not advisable. They point out that even Dr Dukan himself warns of side effects, such as a lack of energy, constipation and bad breath. Wow, those are some great selling points!

The Dukan Diet has millions of followers but every year, the BDA states this is a diet to be avoided for the good of your health. This is though is not the craziest diet, there are some that beggar belief.

Alcorexia: This is where people heavily restrict what they eat during the day, so they can save calories and drink more alcohol without gaining weight. The BDA says, 'To do this in order to 'bank' your calories so you can go a use them on alcohol is pure madness and could easily result in alcohol poisoning and even death'. This is a diet for alcoholics, and yes it really exists!

The Blood Group diet: This diet restricts what people can eat based on their blood group. Its premise is that only certain blood groups can handle certain foods. The BDA says the diet 'is completely based on pseudo-science' and could lead to serious nutrient deficiencies.

The Raw Food Diet: As its name suggests, this diet focuses on eating food raw but also on eating only unpasteurised dairy products. Although some vegetables are more nutritious when eaten raw, the BDA points out many nutritious foods cannot be eaten at all, and it carries a risk of food poisoning.

The Baby Food diet: This diet calls for people to eat up to 14 jars of puree or baby food each day. The BDA says it is a restrictive diet as baby food provides few calories and lacks fibre or texture. Without chewing on firmer food at meal times, you may be left feeling hungry.

Sian Porter, consultant dietitian and spokesperson for the BDA, says, "Sadly, there is no magic wand you can wave. If you have some weight you need to lose, then do it in a healthy, enjoyable and sustainable way. In the long term, this will achieve the results you are after."

These are just five of what I call MFI diets (made for idiots), but sadly, there are many more out there. You would have to be completely off your rocker to think that not eating and drinking in order to consumer excessive amounts of alcohol is either good for you or going to lose your weight. The problem is, in this day and age, if people read something in the newspaper and it is associated with a celebrity, then it gains credibility, no matter how ridiculous it is. There is no need to join the MFI club. I will show you how to lose weight easily and enjoy plentiful, fresh, and nutritious food.

PLEASE DON'T EVER...

If you have ever felt the need to resort to radical solutions to lose weight, or if you have purchased diet pills or anything as crazy, then never give these a second thought again. These are not worth the risk and don't work. Never, ever buy anything off the internet. The risk isn't worth it. I fully appreciate the desperation that drives people to try anything, but is it worth dying for?

Sadly, in April 2015, a young woman died after taking pills purchased on the internet. They contained a highly-toxic substance, known as Dinitrophenol, or DNP. This poisoned her, and she literally burned from the inside. Such a tragic waste. You don't need to resort to extreme tactics, because with the Freshplan you have the POWER.

You don't need to expose yourself to the risk of surgery either. The clinics will tell you it is perfectly safe but there are risks. Also, you are increasing the risks of complications in later life by taking away some of your insides. Like I said before, I am not a doctor but there are risks in going under the knife. No matter how big you are, you can lose weight naturally and change your life.

"It's never too late to be the person you always wanted to be."
George Eliot (adapted)

DON'T GET COMPLACENT

Week by week, the weight will come off. It will be quite a lot for the first couple of weeks. Certainly, after the first week your body will shed a lot of water and correct itself and, for the next few weeks, you will see some sizable chunks of weight come off. There is a danger that you can become complacent, but the moment you do, you will pay the price.

Below is my weight loss progress. You will notice, when I got to 18 stone, I actually put on weight. This is because I got complacent and didn't do all the things I had been doing. I went off plan.

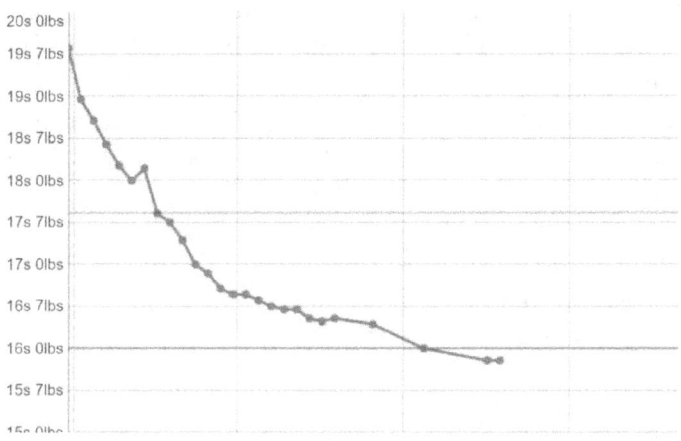

You will encounter natural plateaus in your weight loss. You may find your weight hardly changes for a couple of weeks, even if you have rigidly stuck to your plan.

During the first few weeks, you lose weight fast, primarily because when you reduce your calorie intake, your body releases its stores of glycogen, a type of carbohydrate found in the muscles and liver. As glycogen contains water, the loss of that water has a big impact on your overall body mass. One way to kick start weight loss when you hit a plateau is to step up the exercise and do all you can to speed up your metabolism.

This is a dangerous point when you hit a plateau. Your goblin has the all the ammunition it needs to get you to say sod-it. You may feel you are sticking to the plan, working hard and you are not losing weight. But you will. You must keep going.

I encountered this exact scenario. I hit 18 stone (from 19st 10lb) and stayed there for a couple of weeks. I didn't think I could break through that barrier and got complacent. I said sod-it a couple of times and at the end of a week I had undone plenty of the work I had done. It was a mistake and I learned from my mistake. I deliberately didn't weigh myself for two weeks, I did everything by the book and, as you can see, I broke through and kept the progress going.

I could very easily have gone back to my old ways. Similarly, when you do lose a good amount of weight, you can get complacent because you think you can now lose weight on demand. But your Mindset switches back to the old ways. You must not waiver from the plan and you must get to your target weight by following your plan and not deviating. It is like pedalling a bike up a mountain. It is hard work but when you stop, it is much harder work to get going again, so much so, the momentum has stopped and you might not have the strength to get started again.

Be on your guard for complacency and if you hit a plateau, recognise it for what it is, a natural occurrence. However, do not use this an excuse. Hitting a plateau doesn't mean you will not put weight on if you go off plan, because you will.

Chapter 13
Alcohol and weight loss

Until you reach your target weight, you should abstain completely from alcohol. You may really enjoy a drink, either at home or socially, maybe even both. Alcohol is a no-go. This may horrify you and, if it does, I am sorry but giving it up until you hit your target weight will do you the world of good, and I would argue is essential to your future wellbeing.

First, I am going to declare that I don't drink. Not because I am a recovering alcoholic, nor because I am on a crusade to rid the world of the evils of drink. I just stopped drinking for health reasons and completely lost the inclination to have a drink.

The thought of a hangover or being drunk now makes me wonder why I ever drank in the first place. But I used to enjoy a drink and a night out like everyone else, so I understand the pleasure having a drink brings. But to truly be in control of your weight and your consumption decisions, you need to make the decision to give it up, at least until you achieve your weight loss objective.

According to alcohol concern, more than 9 million people in England drink more than the recommended daily limits. That is just England, not the UK as a whole. That statistic represents around 38 percent of men and 29 percent of women.

Most of those people would not describe themselves as alcoholics but what is an alcoholic? I do not want to get bogged down in what is a massive debate, not least, because I am not qualified to do so. However, I would put forward the case to you that if you are not able to commit and actually stop drinking for a significant period of time, then you have a problem. This may sound like a harsh statement but, in my view, if you cannot stop yourself from drinking then you are addicted. By definition, addiction to alcohol is alcoholism. Alcohol addiction is at the lower end of the spectrum, which progresses to alcohol dependency.

The Daily Mail estimates that one out of every four people in the UK fall under the term, binge drinker. These are people of all ages who consume a large amount of alcohol within a short period of time. People just like getting drunk. I am not going to preach, but alcohol is really bad for you and makes you fat. I think you already know that!

If the prospect of not drinking for several months horrifies you, then you should ask yourself if you have a problem. If so, then you should seek help. I will now explain why you should abstain from all alcohol consumption, at least, until you hit your target weight.

I do not plan to go into detail about alcohol being fattening. I do not want to insult your intelligence. But the key thing here is wine, beer and in fact, most alcoholic drinks are high in calories but they are empty calories. The calories you consume in alcohol are useless to your body. It will simply put weight on you.

Alcohol also leads to mental impairment (shock horror). Again, I know you know this but even one or two drinks, especially if you have not had a drink in a while, will affect your thinking. The

Freshplan is based on your ability to control your thought processes and booze will significantly lower your defences.

Alcohol will stimulate hunger and food cravings. It lessens the inhibitions and the goblin can easily take over and run amok. Everyone I know is the same as I used to be. You have a few drinks then you go for a curry, kebab, burger and sod-it mode kicks in. Even consumed in moderation, alcohol is proven to stimulate appetite. It is actually easier to quit than cut down.

With a high refined sugar content, booze is a big problem. We have discussed the problems associated with excess sugar consumption but there is a danger of consequential sweet cravings arising even through modest alcohol consumption.

A medium glass of wine contains the same amount of calories and sugar as a large slice of Victoria sponge. A pint of cider is equivalent to eating one sugar doughnut. When you put it in those terms, it makes perfect sense why it will hinder your weight loss.

It is not just the calories, the sugar and the poor nutritional value of alcohol that make it a no-go whilst you get to your target weight. It is primarily the effect alcohol has on the brain, which makes it so dangerous. You need to decide what is more important; alcohol and continuing to drink, or achieving your weight loss objectives and goals.

It will be a good test for you and your relationship with alcohol to give it up, at least while you achieve your goals. I am not trying to be a killjoy but I want you to hit your target, and I will say the benefits you will get from a sustained period of abstinence will make the sacrifice worthwhile. It is easy to say, but I guarantee it is probably the safest bet I will ever make.

I have written, in some detail, the need to keep yourself hydrated, so make water your drink. Have sparkling water when you go out; with ice and lemon, it looks like a gin and tonic. But it doesn't matter what it looks like. You don't have to justify yourself to anyone. For me, it was hard at first, being with people who drink but as with everything, it gets easier as time goes by until it becomes the norm.

When you have alcohol cravings, treat them no differently than you do food cravings. Use POWER and I would strongly suggest avoiding situations where you will be more at risk to giving in to your cravings. Take it one day at a time, plan ahead, and stay focused on your objectives and goals.

Reality check: There is no point in embarking on any meaningful weight loss programme if you consume alcohol regularly. If you cannot make the commitment to give up, your issue is probably more with alcohol than food. There is no magic wand to wave to circumvent this. Alcohol and weight loss are not compatible. If you need help with alcohol then visit www.drinkaware.co.uk.

I had an extended discussion with a friend of mine about the Freshplan standpoint on alcohol. His view was we run the danger of alienating people by taking a militant view of alcohol. My view is there is no point in misleading anyone. Of course, in an ideal world of healthy existence and wellbeing, you wouldn't drink at all, but this is the real world.

If you like a drink, then it must be moderated, otherwise you will slip into your old ways. If alcohol was a key reason you became overweight, you will know. The advice we have to give you is that you are better off without alcohol. If would be great if it didn't have detrimental effects, but it does, and that will never change!

Chapter 14
Exercise and lose weight

Exercise is a dirty word to many. Here is the bottom line. You can lose weight, get to your objectives and meet your goals without embarking on a hard-core workout regime. I have already advised that by making sure you move more by clocking-up 10k steps daily, you will do well. But, there is always a 'but', you cannot get physically fitter, faster and stronger, or toned without exercise.

I used to say that people who exercised were crazy and I would say exercise was bad for you, leading to injuries and even the possibility of it killing me. That is a load of rubbish. Exercise, as part of a structured and modified plan, is good for you. Of course, it is good for you. Anyone who says it isn't, except a Doctor if you have a genuine medical issue, is talking crap. What is more, they are doing nothing more than excusing their own sedentary existence.

The single biggest reason people do no exercise is they 'Can't Be Bothered' (#CBB). I spent many years living amongst this group. Though, when I was young, I played sport non-stop and loved it. I knew there was a correlation between no longer being active and becoming a #CBB on my weight. But I ignored that and had another biscuit. It doesn't matter how much or how little you do. You can only experience good things by adding exercise to your life.

The reason most people do not exercise is they are dominated by their chimp brain, which wants to avoid the pain of exertion. It is easy to be a #CBB. I can confirm from personal experience the first step hurts the most, the second a bit less and the pain decreases until you actually start enjoying it. This is the law of diminishing returns. Exercising regularly will completely transform your Mindset. You will feel like a winner and you will start thinking like a winner.

If you want more energy, exercise will deliver it for you in spades. Again, any level of exercise you undertake will contribute to the marginal gains of weight loss.

The UK government advises us to do at least two and a half hours of moderate activity, such as gardening, dancing or brisk walking, or 75 minutes of vigorous exercise, including playing sport, running or aerobics, every week. There are 10,080 minutes in a week. 75 minutes represents less than 1% of your week. Your return, by way of benefits, on time invested is huge.

A brisk daily walk of just 20 minutes could add years to your life, according to a study by Cambridge University. They said lack of exercise killed twice as many people as obesity, and even a modest amount of activity prolonged life. And the least fit had the most to gain. Even a 20 minute walk every day (hit your 10k steps) will be a huge benefit.

Professor Nick Wareham, director of the Medical Research Council epidemiology unit at Cambridge University (who conducted the study), was quoted in the Daily Mail:

"Helping people to lose weight can be a real challenge, and whilst we should continue to aim at reducing population levels of obesity, public health interventions that encourage people to make small but achievable changes in physical activity can have significant health benefits and may be easier to achieve and maintain."

The key words there are 'small and achievable'. I am not advocating a Mo Farrah like training regime, but if you presently do little or no exercise, you will benefit from getting off the sofa and doing something. Do something you enjoy. For me, it is cycling. I love it. I am training for a 10k run. I don't love it but I am determined to reach a personal goal and I do get a great buzz from improving as I work towards it. There will be something you can do, whether it is team sports, keep fit class, or even a few sessions in the gym. I am astonished by how many members of health clubs pay monthly fees and never attend. That is just plain ridiculous.

When you exercise, your body releases chemicals called endorphins. I am sure you have heard of endorphins. They are not reserved for muscled-up gym bunnies. They are waiting for you too. These endorphins interact with the receptors in your brain that reduce your perception of pain. We have spoken about keystone habits. Well, exercise is right at the top of the list. It is what I would term an optional extra on the Freshplan menu. The benefits are too great to ignore. It has to be a no brainer, doesn't it? Excuses on a postcard. I remember what my Dad used to tell me; you can kid others, but you can't ever kid yourself.

I will not bore you with what you already know; you will get fit through exercise. No, you know that Sherlock! Improved self-esteem is a key psychological benefit of regular physical activity. If you feel good, you present a positive aura to others and, as a result, good things can happen. You feel happy and when you feel happy, as already described, there is a positive domino effect on your life.

Endorphins are said to trigger a positive feeling in the body, similar to that of morphine. The feeling that follows a run or workout is often described as 'euphoric', at least it does when you have got your breath back. Research conclusively proves that regular exercise can:

- Reduce stress
- Ward off anxiety and feelings of depression
- Boost self-esteem
- Improve sleep
- Increase sex drive
- As well as multiple physiological benefits

The case for doing exercise is compelling. The hardest part is starting. You will not want to start, and you will dread it, fear it, and completely hate the thought of it. You can come up with plenty of excuses. The one I hear all the time is, I don't have the time. I like to wait a few minutes and ask that person if they watched a particular TV show. Soaps are a great example. EastEnders is on an average of two hours a week, amazing how they always find time for that!

"A 30 minute workout is 2% of your day!"
Carl Harris

How does the 'no time' excuse stack up now? It doesn't. Ask yourself, what harm it can do to give it a go? You might like it. There is a great quote I saw at the gym:

"Winners find a way, losers find an excuse."
Anon

The only thing holding you back is you. Your chimp brain is programmed to avoid pain and anything that exerts stress and uses energy. We imagine things to be far worse than they actually are. What is the worse than can happen? You don't like it then don't do it again. But there is a chance you will actually like it. I always think it is fair to go with the three strikes rule. Try something new three times; if you don't like it, three strikes and it is out! I was once told that the people who feel the most pain are the ones who try the hardest to avoid it. Just a thought!

As I said, it is purely an optional extra, but it is a great way of keeping your mind sharp and generating positive energy. It will also accelerate your weight loss and it will just make you feel better. Maybe not the morning after your first workout but the benefits are without question. It is your choice and, if you decide not to, you will still hit your objectives and goals. Start small - any exercise is better than none. Go at your own pace; there is no pressure. And don't worry about how you think you will look to others in the gym. The truth is, no-one cares. They are so focused or exhausted to give you a second thought.

In the gym, I realised there are two ways to look at people. There is a guy at the gym, who is always there, he is retired, in his sixties and he looks as fit as a fiddle. I can't keep up with him (yet!). I was initially envious of him but envy is a negative emotion and it is effectively jealousy. But why should I be jealous? He hasn't won the lottery. He has worked for his fitness and rather than look at him enviously, I look upon him as a motivational role model. I would love to look that good and be in his shape in 20 years' time. Actually, I'd like to right now! When I started talking to him, he offered so much advice and support, a classic example of how positive emotions bring positivity to your life.

EXERCISE IS GREAT FOR STRESS RELIEF

Stress is one of the worst things that effects our modern day lives. Stress is now known as a major health disorder, affecting millions of people. It is a fact there is a direct link between stress and nutrition. Someone with a healthy and balanced diet is likely to be far less stressed than someone with a poor diet. Stress can have detrimental effects on human physical and mental health.

As well as short term memory loss, bad temper, lack of motivation, poor sleep, lethargy, stress can greatly decrease your sex drive and even cause erectile dysfunction. Stress weakens your immune system, making you susceptible to illness, and it places great strain on your heart, and those are just some of what is a very long list.

Stress is also an emotional trigger for eating. If you are under stress, you will experience greater food cravings and your mental state will be such that you will fall prey to them. So many people have stressful jobs, lives or both that it is important to reduce the impact of stress as much as possible. Okay, this is easier said than done, but if you speak to a clinical psychologist, they say stress can escalate to depression, and the line between stress and mild depression is blurred. You do not want to ever have to take any medication for stress, anxiety or depression. Once you are on them, you are hooked and getting off them can be hell on earth.

Any doctor, councillor or clinical psychologist (worth their salt) will tell you that sleep, exercise and nutrition are the best things to deal with and prevent stress. Exercise stimulates serotonin and other feel good hormones in the brain, which are more powerful than any man made drug. You will have more energy, which will make you feel stronger. This will also lead to better sleep. Whilst you are exercising, you are not thinking about the stuff that gets you stressed, so it is a great distraction and you can also release that frustration and aggression.

A friend of mine works in an office, where everyone is almost always stressed, due to the job they do. I advised them to do some boxing training. It has been so effective the company now pays a coach to hold a weekly session for the office and everyone who attends says it is a huge help. Okay, so this study isn't going to make it into The Lancet but whilst it isn't scientific, if people say it works for them, then it is job done. The point is, the evidence is there and you don't need to be a scientist to work out that getting off your arse and doing some exercise is good for your mind and body.

I said at the start you can look at losing weight as an investment in yourself and those who love you. The same principle applies to exercise. Are you still a #CBB now?

"To keep the body in good health is a duty, otherwise, we shall not be able to keep our mind strong and clear."
Buddha

One final point, hit your target weight and be active, exercising regularly, you can maintain your weight through exercise and you can have some big rewards for doing it. I am doing about 60 miles a week on the bike at the moment. I have no worries about going out for a meal and having a desert because I am burning it off on the road and feel great. The best of both world beckons!

But there is one big reason to exercise. It produces energy and there is nothing more important than energy. The biggest determinant of a happy life, without question in my view, is the level of energy you are able to produce.

Chapter 15
Freshplan: The PELOS concept (Personal Energy Level Output for Success)

The biggest influence on the direction your life takes is what we call the PELOS CONCEPT. In short, this stands for *PERSONAL ENERGY LEVEL OUTPUT [for] SUCCESS*. There is nothing that dictates your motivation, wellbeing and Mindset more than your energy levels.

Energy is the fuel that powers all humans. Every aspect of your existence needs energy. You cannot have enough of it. Many of the issues a human faces on a daily basis is caused by a lack of personal energy level output. Energy powers change and change powers success.

There is a direct correlation between your personal energy levels and the level of success you will have in all areas. Energy powers your physical movement, of course, but it does so much more. Your mental agility, alertness, and all your thought processes are powered by energy.

Your mood is primarily determined by energy too. If you have high energy levels, you will feel better, which as we know has a significant knock-on effect in other areas of your life.

There are three elements to maximise your PELOS. These are categorised as:

- **Eat Well (Good diet)**
- **Live Well (Positive Mindset and habits)**
- **Exercise Well (Generates energy)**

The better you do within each of these areas, the higher your personal energy levels will be. This is a very simple concept and is indeed common sense, but you would be surprised how many people really struggle with energy levels. If your energy is too low, you will know. You may be tired at the end of the day and spend your evenings on the sofa watching TV. You may lack motivation to do the things you know you should do, and you may find it hard to get out of bed in the morning. Improving the three key PELOS determinants, your life will improve exponentially as a result.

I am not sure if this is an academic theory, but I have seen huge *consequential changes* in my life after making changes to my weight, health and ongoing lifestyle. There is no question that I am a much stronger person, both in my physical wellbeing and mind. Positivity breeds, like the proverbial rabbit.

Your journey through life encounters adversity, some more than others. These are obstacles to be negotiated and with an abundance of positive energy, you can deal with them much easier than you ever thought possible. Earlier this year, my personal life was turned upside down.

My mother-in-law died and, almost simultaneously, my own mother was diagnosed with stage 4 breast cancer. A hugely difficult period and all the small daily problems life holds became magnified. I swear the old me would have crumpled. I have had smaller problems than this in the past (that now pale in significance), which I allowed to derail me. It is easy to say that with the benefit of hindsight but this year has proved to me, without any doubt, the consequential changes which have resulted from the changes I have made, make me able to deal with anything life throws at me, better than I ever would. Adversity requires huge amounts of energy. Thankfully I had it when I needed it. You too will have a reservoir of energy to call on should the need arise.

Look at it logically. When we have energy, life is good, we feel good, and we feel happy. When we have no energy, we are tired, down and life is anything but good. People, who are successful, have an abundance of energy. I challenge you to name a winner, or someone successful, who you would categorise as having low energy levels. If you are despondent with low energy, when you are facing adversity, you are much less likely to conquer it. Start investing in energy for the future. It will be the best investment you ever made, guaranteed!

ENERGY POWERS CHANGE

The greatest fuel for powering change is your PERSONAL ENERGY LEVEL OUTPUT. We have talked a lot about vicious cycles but the energy cycle of life is the complete opposite. Once you seek change and start to generate more energy, life becomes a perpetual circle of positivity. Energy creates more energy. Adversity becomes manageable. Success becomes possible.

The motivation, drive and fortitude to power your willpower and your inner drive will all come from the energy you create by the changes detailed by the Freshplan. Eating a healthy diet will increase energy and you will have an immediate benefit from it in all areas of your life. This change will make you live better, employ smarter techniques and be more positive and motivated. This is perpetual as it creates yet more energy. By adding an element of exercise to this, your energy levels will go into the overdrive zone and this is what will power a much more successful life.

When your energy levels dip, it opens the door to sod-it mode. Keeping energy levels high is your defence against giving into your chimp brain and your goblin. You are at your most vulnerable when energy levels dip. Remember this, consistency of effort requires motivation and self-discipline. The more energy you have, the greater your chance of success. Achieving your objectives and goals is just the start.

CHANGE POWERS SUCCESS

With your energy level meter constantly in the overdrive zone, you will find that your life goes into overdrive. Success will not stop at meeting your weight loss and personal health-related goals. You will also start to power success in all other areas of your life. Personal, social business, and relationship success is driven by energy. You should not limit the benefits of the Freshplan to losing weight and keeping it off. You can use the Freshplan for lifelong success. That is the subject of the follow-up. Once you have a Freshplan Mindset, there will be no stopping you.

It is time to start! To make a change, you need to take action and do things differently from what you have done in the past. Reading, learning and agreeing is not enough. We can all offer excuses why we can't start this right now. Those who delay, usually do so indefinitely, and usually never get round to it. Death comes to us all. I plan to delay that as long as possible, but when that point comes, I do not want to realise I had other things to do, which were more important than doing everything I could to delay death.

You can't change the world, but you can change YOUR world. The truest statement you can possibly ever hear is that today is the first day of the rest of your life. You can determine the path the rest of your life takes. You have the Power to live the life and become the person you always aspired to be, fuelled by your personal energy output.

Abraham Harold Maslow was an American psychologist, who was best known for creating Maslow's hierarchy of needs, a theory of psychological health, predicated on fulfilling innate human needs in priority, culminating in self-actualisation. His pyramid is wheeled out regularly in business seminars, but he hit the nail on the head when he said:

"If you deliberately plan on being less than you are capable of being, then I warn you that you'll be unhappy for the rest of your life....In order for you

*to become truly happy that which you can become,
you must become."*
Abraham Maslow

My Grandad always said I could be anything I wanted and I must live life on my own terms. His story is an amazing one but he always said life is very short and can pass you by if you choose to sit on the side-lines and be a mere observer. Fulfilment is the key to happiness, and to live life to the fullest, you need energy. Happiness comes from within, success is achieved not awarded and, above all, change happens only by design. Personal Energy Level Output delivers Success. Change delivers consequential changes to your life. Take care of your Personal Energy Levels that will power your life. The more energy you have, the better life becomes.

You need to be in good shape and full of energy to be the person you want to be. You have one life, only one, but you have a second chance, starting right now to live it the way you want. You have already stated, at least in part, the person you want to be, a thinner healthier version of you. You have the power to become that person, so it is time to start the journey from failure to success, from despair to lifelong happiness.

Part Two:

THE FRESHPLAN PELOS DIET

Eat Well, Live Long and Prosper

Chapter 16
Freshplan: Introducing the Freshplan PELOS Diet

The big news is that everything we are and everything we do is powered by energy. Energy comes from food. Whatever you want to achieve in life requires energy. From the basics of human existence to success in every aspect of life, it all requires energy. The more energy you have, the better your life is. Health, Wealth and Happiness all require energy. The only goals that energy will not achieve for you are not ones you ever want to realise.

I do not want to overcomplicate things. The PELOS DIET is the complete opposite of complicated. It is the easiest diet known to man because it is the diet that mankind is designed to eat. **PELOS** stands for Personal Energy Level Output for Success. Energy powers life.

I regard everyday as one where I can go out on a spending spree. My currency is positive energy and I throw it around like the fabled Rockefellers. Having a bottomless pit to delve into makes life great and spending it a pleasure. I am living my life, my way. I want you to start doing exactly the same.

I have called the Freshplan Diet the PELOS diet because as well as losing weight, you will have so much more energy, possibly than you can ever remember. Weight loss diets are notoriously complicated to follow and involve you fasting and eating stuff you don't enjoy. I have deliberately created a plan, which is none of those things. This is so simple you will wonder why you have never done it before. It is so effective you will eat like this for the rest of your life.

So what is the Freshplan PELOS Diet? You are no doubt anxious to find out! The modern diet (not weight loss plan) is based on manufactured food, which is high in sugar, fat, salt and lots of additives that mess with our mind and body. Food has been so artificially produced the average human now does not get anywhere close to the natural nutrients the body needs.

The human body is an amazing thing and you will be amazed at its ability to heal and reset itself. All you have to do is fuel your body with what it needs. I am amazed by how much people spend on skin and hair treatments when all they actually have to do is eat right. Manufactured food may look great, smell great, and taste unbelievably amazing, but it can't come close to fulfilling nature's job. The PELOS diet takes us back to nature and a diet based on natural fresh food.

Ah, the caveman diet! I can hear you screaming you have heard it all before. Well, if you want to eat like a caveman, be my guest. They lived until they were about 25, ate what they could get, were under nourished and died of the most basic of bacterial infection. Fortunately, we have evolved a long way, and as a species, we have knowledge of nutrition and access to a plentiful supply of food from around the world.

Our bodies have an amazing ability to make you feel good, look good, get healthy and fight off many of the things that repeatedly get us down and make us feel bad. The problem is, to do this, it needs the right fuel to do it. We have over-evolved and we are bypassing nature's food chain when it comes to nutrition. By eating a staple diet that is fresh food based, you will free yourself from the toxic effects that some manufactured food has on you and improve the quality of your nutrient intake by a massive amount.

So how does eating natural food help me lose weight? I'm sure that's what you're thinking! Well, good question and quite easy to answer. When you take out all the rubbish from your diet (I am using the vernacular for simplicity), your body will start working as it should. It is not natural for humans, like wild animals, to be fat. Forget domesticated animals for a moment and think of animals, mice, squirrels, foxes, lions, tigers, in fact, you name it; wild animals are not fat.

They eat what they instinctively know they should eat, eat only when they are hungry and eat what they need. This all sounds great in an ideal world but we don't live in one and we are not living in the wild. Hunter-gathering skills for the human extend to finding a parking space at the supermarket and being expert in plastic bag packing.

The point I am making is this: if you flip your diet from one dominated by processed food and low in natural nutrients to one that is fresh and natural based, then the majority of your food intake will provide your body with everything it needs to do what it is made to do. Your body will start to work in the way it should, and it will look after you. The change you will feel will be nothing short of miraculous.

For most people living the processed food nightmare, hunger is driven by the brain. I do not think I ever experienced true hunger when I was shovelling in Jaffa Cakes by the packet. Sure, I had food cravings but hunger that comes from the stomach is something I can't recall. Now, I understand how my body really works and am able to regulate consumption in the way my body should. Since I changed to a natural food diet, the one thing I do not miss is that constant bloated feeling, always eating until I was full. I used to be a constant gas bag, a danger to the environment, Mr Methane, but no longer. I am no Gillian McKeith, the famous TV personality who examined peoples' diets, but suffice to say, everything works as it should, regular as clockwork. The one thing you will learn is that your body, if you let it, works just fine.

I said at the start of this book, I am not advocating extreme diets or becoming a health preacher. I still eat processed foods, and yes, the odd Jaffa Cake passes my lips, but these are treats, not my staple diet. You must give your body what it needs to work properly.

If you bought a brand new car, you wouldn't start putting in cooking oil when it needs diesel. It may get you from A-to-B but it wouldn't do so smoothly, and you would be doing irreversible damage to the engine and systems. Your body is the most valuable thing you own, yet we are doing exactly the same thing to ourselves.

Human beings can't function as they should by living on a manufactured food diet. 'Five-a-day' is a slogan everyone has become familiar with. The reality is, five a day is a bare minimum needed to survive. According to The World Health Organisation, 2.7 million deaths would be avoided annually worldwide if everybody ate 400g of fruit and vegetables a day.

In 2008, the government stated that lower than recommended intake of fruit and vegetables was to blame for 42,200 premature deaths annually in the UK and poor nutrition has cost the NHS £6bn in treatment and care. I am not sure if that £6bn is included in the £9bn that Type 2 diabetes costs the NHS, but I think the point is crystal clear. Fresh food is the food of life.

Everything that is good for us is found in fresh food. For example, polyphenols in apples and berries are good for cancer prevention, as are green leafy vegetables. Garlic and onions are high in prebiotics, which stimulate gut bacteria and are good for the bowel.

Fresh food is full of antioxidants, which help your body thrive and fend off disease and bacteria. The list is endless and, for whatever reason, humans have decided the stuff that keeps us alive, makes us live longer, and makes us feel great is something we no longer want to eat. Five a day in the UK is advised but in France the number is 10, and in Japan 17 a day is recommended. What the message should be is fresh food is what you are built to eat, and fresh food will solve many of the health issues of the world.

Certainly, obesity, which is a worldwide epidemic, would not be a problem if humans feasted on proper food. That word proper food was not slipped in there by accident. Fresh food, natural food, call it what you like, is proper food. Manufactured food is not proper food. Humans are now under nourished and are following a diet that is toxic to our physiology. Not only that, manufactured food not only causes our physical systems to breakdown but it impairs our psychology, preventing us from controlling the WWW (What, When and Why) of what we eat. I contend the five a day message is nothing short of a delusion. Sure, five a day is better than nothing, but it is nowhere near enough.

Eating five a day as part of a diet that is full of sugar, processed fat and foods lacking in nutritional value will have very little beneficial long-term impact on the human body. We have lost sight completely of what we need to be eating and why we actually need to eat. Sure, the argument I always get is that food should be enjoyed. I am sure people enjoyed smoking 60 a day but I bet they didn't feel good, look good, function well or even smell great after doing that for a few years.

Someone told me they didn't like the taste of water. The ultimate nonsense. Water has no taste but what they actually meant was I am hooked on artificially produced flavours and now my brain rejects the most basic of human requirements. We are two thirds water. It is impossible for humans to reject water. It is a classic case of a dysfunctional food psychology system.

That is the key. Where systems are dysfunctional, physical and psychological, they can be easily repaired. By eating the right foods, your body will heal itself in no time. Dysfunctional systems often lead to malfunctions, which is when medical attention is required. The good news is your system will start to work perfectly once you start eating the right things and cutting out the nasty stuff.

You will find you have so much more personal energy as a result. A manufactured based diet simply doesn't give you enough of the nutrients you need to meet your physiological requirements and it doesn't provide enough energy. That is why many people feel lethargic and are constantly miserable. It is really simple to change too. Again, it's a simple habit to change.

The most bizarre thing, and I did it for years, is when you go to a supermarket, the first aisles are always the fresh food, fruit and vegetables, and so forth, yet we walk on by and head for the manufactured stuff. Have a look at your final basket of shopping. You may be surprised by just how little fresh food you buy and, consequentially, eat every week.

The more you shift the balance of food towards fresh food, the higher your energy will be. When you start cranking up the energy, you will find the more you have, the more you want. It is far better to be addicted to energy than it ever will be, being addicted to sugar. You just have to break out of that vicious cycle of addiction. It will be easier than you think and once you get in the habit, it will become the norm.

The more good habits and healthy norms you instigate, the better. Once you make it a norm, it will become second nature and written into your personal mindware. I used to reach for the biscuit tin when I was hungry. Now, I turn to the fruit bowl, which is always fully stocked. I made a decision to switch from full fat milk to semi-skimmed a few years ago, soon after full fat milk became objectionable. When I decided to lose weight, I did the same thing, this time to skimmed milk.

At first, I thought it tasted like water but it quickly became the norm, and now I can't abide anything else. The point is, your first reaction to healthy change is not always, indeed rarely is, your enduring one. I have not found any scientific theory to validate this but I have found it happens time and time again.

I have also found some hard truths, sadly, a few years later than I would like. There are foods you simply have to eat that don't appeal as much as the foods you really want to eat. But there is a payoff and the mother of all lessons is there is a payoff for everything you do.

The payoff can be good or bad, but it is almost always known when making your choices. If you want to live it up, feast on sugar, junk food and generally focus on taste not nutrition, then that is your choice, but the payoff is, as you know, being fat and unhealthy with low energy levels. You have to decide which you want more. Of course you want both, but in the real world, it isn't possible. When you look at it objectively, there is no decision to make. Sure a taste sensation tastes great, but how long does it last? A few moments at best. Looking good, feeling good, and doing good is more enjoyable and lasts much longer. Energy rules.

The PELOS diet is a different way to eat, but it is the right way to eat. It will redress your energy shortages. It does not mean you never eat anything but fresh food for the rest of your life, but it does mean you will focus on giving your body what it needs and stop living a toxic existence. You will kick the sugar and junk food addiction, and if you are worried about cold turkey, don't be. Turkey is a great source of protein!

The PELOS DIET is in three phases:

- **PHASE ONE: The 7-day detox turbo fat burner**
- **PHASE TWO: Getting to your target weight**
- **PHASE THREE: On-going weight management**

Let's get started!

Chapter 17
Phase 1: The 7-day detox fat burner

> **IMPORTANT:** *If you have any medical conditions or you are taking medication, please consult your Doctor before embarking on this, or any, weight loss plan. If you suffer from diabetes, you MUST speak to your doctor before embarking on this plan. You may need to skip to phase 2 if your doctor advises.*

This is where your Freshplan journey starts. It is now time to start losing weight. The '7-day detox turbo fat booster' is optional but I highly recommend doing it. For the next seven days, you will follow a diet consisting of only fresh fruit and vegetable smoothies and drinking plenty of water.

These are highly nutritious and will clean your system, give you a massive energy boost and start to burn fat. I would expect you to lose seven pounds in the next seven days.

We are going straight into it for the next seven days. Of course, there is no alcohol permitted and I would strongly suggest you do not drink tea or coffee either for the next seven days. Only water and only water can be consumed after 7pm. The first thing to say is this is not a quick-fix. We are doing this to reboot your system, get your body back in tune with its natural functions and clear out the toxins.

You will need a blender. There is no need to spend too much. I bought one for about £25 from Amazon and it does everything I need. I use it twice a day, sometimes more. It works a treat.

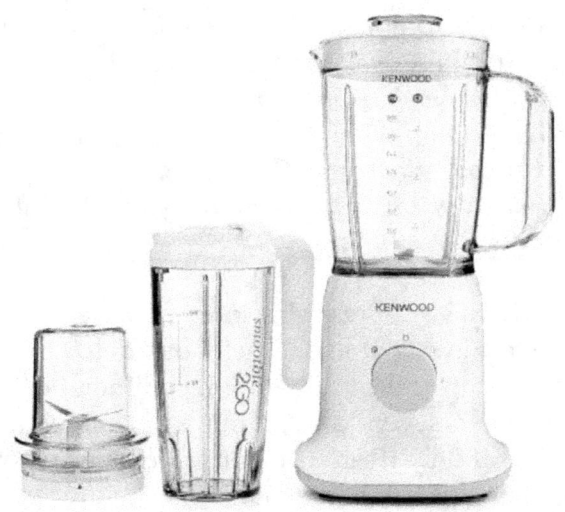

The plan is to have FOUR smoothies every day. I do not advocate juicing. I am a firm believer in blending or smoothie making. If you are only juicing fruits, this would cause a rapid spike in blood sugar and unstable blood sugar levels can lead to mood swings, energy loss, memory problems and more!

The blending process breaks the fibre apart (which makes the fruit and vegetables easier to digest), but also helps create a slow, even release of nutrients into the bloodstream and avoids blood sugar spikes. Smoothies tend to be more filling because of the fibre, not to mention they are much easier and quicker to make.

I have put together a shopping list for the suggested smoothies but I would like to make a very important point. As long as you stick to the golden rule, only add fresh fruit and vegetables and have at least one PELOS GREEN POWER SMOOTHIE a day, you can make your own recipes. Remember, do not go off plan and do not add anything other than fresh food, and absolutely NO sugar or sweeteners. The first smoothie of the day needs to be a PELOS GREEN POWER SMOOTHIE.

Start each day with a probiotic tablet and glass of water. As soon as you get up, your first job always is to hydrate and take your good bacteria.

WATER: STAY HYDRATED AT ALL TIMES!

To be fully hydrated, adults need to take on 1.5ml of water for every calorie burned, which means you need a minimum of 3 litres of water each day. Water fills you up, keeps you hydrated and helps burn fat. Do not take on any liquid calories; only water is permitted to drink. Sparkling water is perfectly acceptable.

The next pages have the 7 Day Detox Power Smoothie Schedule.

THE 7 DAY DETOX POWER SMOOTHIE SCHEDULE

Supplements	Breakfast	Mid-morning	Early afternoon	Before 7pm
DAY 1 Probiotic tablet	PELOS GREEN POWER SMOOTHIE (1)	THE BLACK AND BLUE (2)	ORANGE CARROT AND GINGER (11)	THE PINA COLADA (3)
DAY 2 Probiotic tablet	PELOS GREEN POWER SMOOTHIE (1)	APPLE BANANA AND STRAWBERRY (4)	ORANGE BANANA AND PINEAPPLE (8)	MANGO AND PASSION FRUIT (5)
DAY 3 Probiotic tablet	PELOS GREEN POWER SMOOTHIE (1)	THE BLACK AND BLUE (2) + STRAWBERRIES	CRANBERRY ORANGE AND APPLE (13)	VANILLA AND HONEY DELIGHT (7)

DAY 4 **Probiotic tablet**	PELOS GREEN POWER SMOOTHIE (1)	APPLE BANANA AND STRAWBERRY (4)	GREEN APPLE AND CINNAMON SMOOTHIE (12)	THE PINA COLADA (3)
DAY 5 **Probiotic tablet**	PELOS GREEN POWER SMOOTHIE (1)	CRANBERRY ORANGE AND APPLE (13)	ORANGE CARROT AND GINGER (11)	MANGO AND NECTARINES (6)
DAY 6 **Probiotic tablet**	PELOS GREEN POWER SMOOTHIE (1)	THE BLACK AND BLUE (2) AND RASPBERRIES	BANANA AND MEDJOOL DATES (13)	ORANGE BANANA AND PINEAPPLE (8) ADD FRESH GINGER (9)
DAY 7 **Probiotic tablet**	PELOS GREEN POWER SMOOTHIE (1)	APPLE BANANA AND STRAWBERRY (4)	GREEN APPLE AND CINNAMON SMOOTHIE (12)	VANILLA AND HONEY DELIGHT (7)

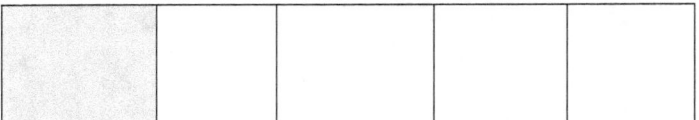

These are the recipes for making the smoothies.

THE PELOS GREEN POWER SMOOTHIE (1)

This is a morning power boost, a glass of nutritional goodness and slow release of proteins to get you started for the day ahead. This will fill you with energy for the day ahead. To make a Green Power Smoothie, add the following:

- 500ml Unsweetened Almond milk or more or less as required for consistency.
- 1x apple, red or green, your choice (add another if you want sweeter taste)
- 1x large banana
- 1x teaspoon of spirulina powder (4g)
- 1 x teaspoon of power greens (optional)
- Add cinnamon (optional)

Obvious statement time, core the apple, do not peel. Take banana out of the skin (derr!) and throw it all in a blender and turn it on. 30 seconds should do it. Put in a glass and serve with ice if preferred. This is such a good way to start the day. You can add anything fresh to this. I sometimes add kiwi fruit or kale. Even garlic. It depends on your palate. The benefit you get from is out of this world. I have added kale, spinach and avocado in the past but these are just optional extras. You can't get enough greens in the morning!

Almond milk you can buy; make sure it is unsweetened. You can make it yourself if you want, but it is far easier to buy it. If you cannot consume almonds due to allergy, then you can use soya, rice or other nut-based milks. They must be unsweetened. Do not use cow's milk of any kind. I use almond milk because it is really nutritious. Soya milk will do if needed but the lowest fat and unsweetened version. Almond milk is the best if you can take it.

Almond milk is really good for you. It has fewer calories than skimmed milk but has zero fat and is high in healthy oils. It is high in vitamins, notably D and E and has absolutely no sugar. It has a very low GI. It has fibre, which aids digestion. If you are lactose intolerant, almond milk is perfectly fine. It has benefits for blood pressure and contains zero, yes zero cholesterol. You will also notice improvement in your skin as a result of almond milk. I stress again; it must be unsweetened with no additives. 500ml of almond milk contains around 65 (good) calories.

Apples are extremely good for you, one of the best things you can eat. You can look up the many benefits of apples, but they give a nice sweet healthy taste to your smoothie. We do not need to write extensively why apples are good for you because an apple a day does keep the doctor away! We have always known that!

Bananas are superb for smoothies. They give you a nice taste, good consistency and a neutral colour. I add bananas to every smoothie I make! They are a superfood but, to be fair, all fresh food is a superfood, compared to manufactured processed food, which is rubbish (in the main). Apples have taken all the glory over the years but bananas are amazingly healthy. Bananas are high in potassium, which reduces blood pressure. I can testify it does. I eat in excess of a dozen a week and my BP has reduced significantly. Bananas also have antacid effects, protecting the stomach from ulcers and their subsequent damage. Best of all, they are loaded with energy, better than any energy bar on the market. They contain high amounts of tryptophan, an amino acid that helps boost serotonin production, which can lead to better moods and a better night sleep.

Spirulina Powder is something you may not have heard of. Spirulina is one of (if not number 1) the most nutritious, complete, efficient, and effective foods on Earth. It is the most concentrated whole food source of protein. Spirulina is 60-70% protein and 83-95% digestible. Spirulina is the most concentrated form of any known organic food. Full of nutritional wonders, it goes beyond superfood. Spirulina has everything you need to live on, more than any other protein, grain, plant, algae, herb, vitamin, and anything! It's so nutritious and digestible that you get all the nutrition in just one level tablespoon (9 grams). The U.N. Industrial Development Organization (UNIDO) commissioned a five-year toxicology study on Spirulina and found it to be a safe, non-toxic food, and in a separate study, it is 'recommended as a potential solution to the world food crisis and global protein shortage.'

Many people use spirulina daily to help naturally detoxify their bodies, maintain a healthy weight, and boost their energy. Studies have shown that spirulina can:

- Help your body fight infection
- Inhibit allergic reactions
- Destroy infected and cancerous cells
- Lower your cholesterol
- Raise your HDL (good cholesterol) levels and lower bad cholesterol levels.
- Give you an energy boost.

This is something you should have every day of your life. You can buy Spirulina capsules, which are far better than any pharmaceutical tablet you can take. If you get a few minutes, look up the nutritional benefits of spirulina on Google. It is mind boggling how this wonder food has been overlooked for so long. Not anymore, you have found a life changing food. Do not overlook the benefits of spirulina. This is an energising food. Spirulina is money well spent.

Power greens is available in health food shops and is made from fresh veg. It is effectively fresh vey extract, concentrated. There are various types available and all will (or should) include spirulina; however, they also include a range of other foods. They can be quite expensive, so shop around on the internet. Make sure you buy UNFLAVOURED ones with no added sugars. I pay £7.99 plus delivery for 100g online. That is 25 teaspoons, 25 days' worth! The more nutrients you take in, the better for you.

Cinnamon is optional if you like the taste but I would strongly advise taking it. Cinnamon may lower blood sugar in people with type 1 or type 2 diabetes, according to Diabetes UK. According to the U.S. National Library of Medicine, cinnamon is used to help treat muscle spasms, vomiting, diarrhoea, infections, the common cold, loss of appetite, and erectile dysfunction (ED). A food that puts lead in your pencil can't be ignored!

The *PELOS POWER GREEN SMOOTHIE* will not look appetizing, at first, but it tastes just fine. However, it is jam-packed with goodness and will give you instant energy. Make sure you have one of these every morning. You will feel the benefit of this. Your personal energy meter will be higher than it has been for a long time. You will feel vibrant and start your day in a better mood.

THE BLACK AND BLUE (1)

This is our take on Ribena. It tastes better and infinitely better for you. You can make this in less than a minute. In 2007, a study conducted by the Australian Consumers' Association for Choice magazine revealed blackcurrant juice (from concentrate) only constituted 5% of the Ribena Fruit Drink product. This is the real thing! You are boosting your health and immunity with the Black and Blue.

- 500ml Unsweetened Almond Milk or more or less as required for consistency.
- 1x handful of blackberries
- 1x handful of blackcurrants
- 1x handful of blueberries

This tastes so good! This is better than anything you can buy, which is full of sugar and chemicals. This packs a super energy punch, and these berries are true superfoods packed with goodness.

Blackberries are much like spinach, raisins, apples, plums and grapes, rich in bioflavonoids and Vitamin C, but other nutritional benefits include a very low sodium. The dark blue colour ensures blackberries have one of the highest antioxidant levels of all fruits. Antioxidants are nature's doctor, fending off disease and boosting your immunity.

Blueberries are marketed as wonder food and contain vitamin C, fibre, manganese and other antioxidants (notably anthocyanins). They taste great too and provide plenty of energy.

Blackcurrants are often overlooked but are great tasting! Blackcurrants are especially rich in Vitamin C - containing more than three times as much as an orange! They can even help prevent joint inflammation, eyestrain and urinary infections, and yes, they are packed with antioxidants.

THE PINA COLADA (3)

This is packed with goodness and tastes out of this world! No alcohol (sadly), but it will feel like you are on your tropical island.

- 500ml of coconut milk, unseated if possible
- Fresh pineapple
- 1 teaspoon of coconut extract
- 1 x banana
- Cinnamon (optional)

Skin the pineapple and slice. Remove banana from skin, put in blender with the coconut milk and teaspoon of coconut extract. Blend. Job done. What a way to end the day.

Pineapple fruit contains a proteolytic enzyme bromelain that digests food by breaking down protein. Bromelain also has anti-inflammatory, anti-clotting and anti-cancer properties. Studies have shown that consumption of pineapple regularly helps fight against arthritis, indigestion and worms. Pineapple is also an excellent source of antioxidants, vitamin C, vitamin A and thiamine, pyridoxine, riboflavin and minerals, like copper, manganese and potassium. Trust me; it is all good stuff. This is a great way to end the day.

APPLE, BANANA AND STRAWBERRY (4)

No fancy name for this one, and no prizes for guessing how to make either.

- 500ml Unsweetened almond milk or more or less as required for consistency.
- 1x handful of strawberries
- 1 x banana
- 1x apple

Core the apple, peel the banana, and remove the green stems from the strawberries. Throw it in the blender and 30 seconds later, there you go. You will never buy a shake from a fast food joint again after you have tasted this!

Strawberries are another superfood and taste great. So many things are artificially flavoured with strawberry, but this is the real thing. Scientific studies show that consumption of these berries may have potential health benefits against cancer, aging, inflammation and neurological diseases. Packed with antioxidants, vitamins and, of course, energy.

MANGO AND PASSION FRUIT (5)

This is terrific. Mango and passion fruits are available in supermarkets. If you do not know how to peel and prepare, type it in to YouTube for lots of quick videos, dead easy! This will give you a sweet, zingy (is that a word?) taste. Full of flavour and energy.

- 500ml Unsweetened almond milk or more or less as required for consistency.
- 1x mango peeled and diced
- 2 x passion fruits (middle not case)
- 1 x banana (peeled)

- 1 x apple (cored)

This will surprise you. It's sensationally good. Tropical taste and not only full or flavour, but full of nutritional goodness.

Mangos have more than 20 vitamins and minerals. Factoid - mangos are the most consumed fruit in the world. They lead to a decreased risk of macular degeneration, a decreased risk of colon cancer, improvement in digestion and bone health and even benefits for the skin and hair. Great source of energy.

Passion fruits are real fruits. They are not heavily consumed in the UK, but they should be. They are a good source of fibre. Full of vitamin A and C. Lots of minerals too. Iron, copper, magnesium and phosphorus are present in adequate amounts in the fruit. Great for your immune system.

MANGO AND NECTARINES (6)

This as above, but with nectarines not passion fruit. This will be very sweet and oh so nice. You will want more of this. I guarantee it. You need to remove the stone from the nectarine. There is no need to peel it, unless you want to but the peel is good for you.

Nectarines are like peaches, but not furry! They are indeed packed with numerous health promoting anti-oxidants, plant nutrients, minerals and vitamins. They are a healthy source of some B-complex vitamins and minerals. It is good in niacin, pantothenic acid, thiamine and pyridoxine. In addition, it contains an appropriate ratio of minerals and electrolytes, such as potassium, iron, zinc, copper and phosphorus. Iron is required for red blood cell formation. Potassium is an important component of cell and body fluids that help regulate heart rate and blood pressure.

VANILLA AND HONEY DELIGHT (7)

This is your treat. You will adore this, my all-time favourite, and it's so good for you.

- 500ml Unsweetened almond milk or more or less as required for consistency
- 2 x bananas
- 1 teaspoon of Manuka honey
- 1 teaspoon or almond extract
- 1x pinch of poppy seeds

Manuka Honey is quite expensive BUT it is a scientific marvel and worth the investment. It's so good at healing infection that in many hospitals around the world now, Active Manuka Honey is used when nothing else works for treatment of antibiotic resistant MRSA super bugs. It will give you an energy boost, a great sweet taste and boost your immune system. One jar will last you a long time. It tastes great too!

Poppy seeds give this a nice flavour and bit of crunch. Poppy seeds contain many plant derived chemical compounds that are found to have anti-oxidant, disease preventing, and health promoting properties. Poppy seeds are high in fibre and contain good levels of minerals, like iron, copper, calcium, potassium, manganese, zinc and magnesium.

ORANGE BANANA AND PINEAPPLE (8)

This is full of vitamins minerals and energy. You must peel the orange of course.

- 500ml Unsweetened Almond Milk or more or less as required for consistency.
- 2 x peeled oranges
- 1 x banana
- 1 x skinned pineapple

Oranges are full of vitamin C and taste great. One of the world's premier flavours, orange juice, but this is all the orange with fibre and all the goodness.

ORANGE BANANA AND PINEAPPLE WITH GINGER (9)

As weird as this sounds, adding fresh ginger will surprise you with the taste. You need to peel the ginger. Again, see YouTube for help if required.

Ginger is among the healthiest (and most delicious) spices on the planet. It is loaded with nutrients and bioactive compounds that have powerful benefits for your body and brain. It is high in gingerol, a substance with powerful anti-inflammatory and antioxidant properties. If you like ginger, you can add this to your breakfast smoothie but this is your choice, depending on taste.

BANANA AND MEDJOOL DATES (10)

This is going to blow your mind. I love this.

- 500ml Unsweetened Almond Milk or more or less as required for consistency.
- 2 x peeled bananas
- 6 x fresh medjool dates
- 1 x teaspoon of almond extract

Dates are sweet but they are very good for you! They are very sweet and packed with energy. This will give you a boost. They are also full of fibre and good for your, err, digestion shall we say. Good for cholesterol and jam-packed with healthy minerals and vitamins. They have high natural sugar, so we don't have them every day!

ORANGE CARROT AND GINGER (11)

You need to peel the carrots and the top and tail. Peel the oranges and ginger too. This is good for you, and you will see in the dark before long.

- 500ml Unsweetened almond milk or more or less as required for consistency.
- 2 x peeled carrots
- 2 x peeled oranges
- 1 x slice peeled ginger

Carrots may sound strange to add to a smoothie but it is really healthy for you. Full of vitamin A and vitamin C. They are also plentiful in carotene that has been proven to help ward off cancer. Always eat your carrots. Even if you don't like them on a plate, you will love them in this sweet smoothie with a kick.

GREEN APPLE AND CINNAMON SMOOTHIE (12)

This is a very healthy smoothie with plenty of goodness, and it tastes great too. Kale is a superfood but use only the leaves.

- 500ml Unsweetened almond milk or more or less as required for consistency
- 2 medium green apples.
- ½ teaspoon of cinnamon
- 1 medium banana
- 1 cup of kale leaf

Kale is full of fibre, which regulates your blood sugar. It is rich in vitamins A, C and K. Lutein and zeaxanthin, nutrients that give kale its deep, dark green colouring and protect against macular degeneration and cataracts. Minerals including phosphorus, potassium, calcium and zinc.

CRANBERRY ORANGE AND APPLE (13)

This tastes amazing and full of energy! Will give you a boost. Really full of good stuff, quick and easy to make.

- 500ml Unsweetened almond milk or more or less as required for consistency
- 2 apples
- 2 oranges
- Handful of cranberries.

Cranberries are good for you. Research studies show that cranberry juice consumption offers protection against gram-negative bacterial infections, such as E.coli in the urinary system by inhibiting bacterial-attachment to the bladder and urethra. In addition, cranberries are also a good source of many vitamins, like vitamin C, vitamin A, ß-carotene, lutein, zeaxanthin, and folate, and minerals, like potassium and manganese.

YOU MUST STICK TO THE PLAN FOR 7 DAYS

You may think there is not enough greens but we pack them in first thing. You are getting well-nourished with your daily greens. You are going to get plenty of energy and burn fat. After seven days, you will feel great.

Portion: you should not exceed a pint glass in volume. Do not come unstuck by snacking on forbidden foods, and certainly, do not drink anything but water.

IMPORTANT: Keep drinking water, lots of water, at least one pint of water before your first smoothie of the day and a minimum of six pints throughout the day. If you feel hungry, have a banana. No more than ONE a day (in addition to smoothies). No food after 7pm, no coffee or tea, just your smoothies and water. Stick with it; it will be worth it.

THE 14 DAY SUPER DETOX TURBO FAT BURNER

This is optional, depending on how you feel. Some people find it easier than others. For me, personally, the energy boost I got and the feel-good factor was immense. You may have found coming off sugar, caffeine or alcohol hard. The body goes through a process of rebooting and you also may go into what is known as ketosis.

Ketosis occurs when the body starts burning fat at an extremely high rate. Even the brain runs on fat via ketone bodies. These are energy molecules in the blood (like blood sugar), which become fuel for our brains after being converted from fat by the liver.

In essence, your body starts using the fat it has stored away, you are losing weight. However, for some people this a process that is easier to deal with than others. I have no issue with it; in fact, I thrive on it. For others, you may have some effects, like headache, nausea, fatigue or bad breath. But don't panic. This will happen for no more than three days. I have not had anyone have any severe effects on the 7-day detox at all, but the point is, if you feel different, this is the reason; you are detoxing, and it works.

If at the end of the seven days you are feeling great, there is no harm in repeating the process for another week. In fact, you will get huge benefits and could lose another seven pounds in weight. Everyone is different, so there is no hard and fast rule regarding weight loss. I call this the Super Detox. I know, I'm a genius on the branding front!

Important: The maximum time advised for living on smoothies only is 14 days. We have a digestive system designed to eat and chew food for a reason, so do not ever exceed 14 days at a time. Of course, you can do the detox from time to time for a boost or to get back on track. I went on holiday, lived it up for a week in five star luxury and put on eight pounds or so. I came home, did the detox and a week later, I was back to normal. **But do not exceed 14 days before moving to phase 2.**

If you do the 14 day Super Detox, you will see amazing results. Your energy will be through the roof, and you will see some significant weight loss. You should physically see a difference and you will be very positive about life.

It is purely optional to extend it by another week but I recommend it at the start of the Freshplan Diet. The PELOS concept kicks in straight away and you have the energy boost to power your success into phase 2, which is to reach your target weight.

7 Day Detox Turbo Fat Burner Shopping List:

- Probiotic tablets, available from health food shops or online.
- Almond milk. Unsweetened. (It is really important you get the unsweetened version)
- Apples (organic if possible)
- Bananas (Fair Trade and organic if possible)

- Power Greens Powder (Holland and Barratt and all health food shops or online via www.theproteinworks.com)
- Spirulina Powder (nothing added) Sevenhills 500g is £13.99 via Amazon.
- Blackberries - fresh
- Blackcurrants - fresh
- Blueberries - fresh
- Pineapple - fresh not tinned
- Coconut milk (unsweetened if available)
- Coconut extract
- Strawberries- Fresh
- Mango- fresh
- Passion fruits- fresh
- Nectarines- fresh
- Vanilla extract
- Manuka Honey (preferable to raw honey)
- Poppy seeds
- Fresh raspberries
- Fresh ginger
- Medjool Dates
- Almond extract
- Fresh Garlic
- Carrots - fresh
- Fresh kale
- Cinnamon
- Cranberries - fresh

For the 14 day Super Detox, do it again! You can mix up the smoothies but make sure you have the breakfast smoothies every day. There is a wider range of smoothie recipes on the Freshplan website at www.freshplan.com.

The Freshplan Diet by Carl Harris

Chapter 18
Phase 2: Getting to your target weight

Following your 7 Day Detox or 14 Day Super Detox, you are ready for Phase 2. You are on the way, the weight is starting to go and you will feel positive, motivated and ready to reach your target. You will have so much more energy and, as we know, energy powers success. Phase 2 is where you go back to eating normally, as in not living purely on smoothies, rather than returning to what was normal for you before. Phase 2 will take as long as is required for you to hit your target weight. Clearly, there is no fixed time because everyone is different.

It is important for me to stress that the rate of weight loss during the initial detox period will not be what you lose every week. It is not healthy for long-term weight loss, i.e. staying slim to crash diet. You will lose weight at a decreasing rate as weeks go by; this is perfectly normal and is indeed perfectly healthy. The Freshplan is designed to not only lose weight but to get you healthy, fill you with energy and do so in a way that sets you up for the long-term.

We are doing things the right way; we are working with nature. I could tell you to just live on smoothies until you get to your target weight. It would be quick but it would not be healthy. Losing weight is important but being healthy is the most important thing. If all you did was the detox plan for weeks and months on end, you would easily put weight on when you went back to eating whole food. The moral of this is to not be tempted to cut corners and keep to the smoothies and ignore the plan. You need to have a healthy balanced diet and get into a routine that will not only get you to your target weight but make sure you stay there for good and you are healthy and well nourished. If you stay on the detox plan indefinitely, you will start to feel low in energy. Trust me, 14 days max, then Phase 2.

I fully understand why some people are tempted just to keep going on smoothies alone and nothing else, but it is unwise and I cannot advocate it in any way. However, fear not; we are not putting away the blender or giving up on the smoothies for good. In fact, they play a huge role in both Phase 2 and Phase 3 of the Freshplan PELOS Diet.

Never lose sight of the fact that energy powers your success, and energy comes primarily from food. It is boosted by exercise.

START SOME EXERCISE

This is the point where I urge you to ensure you are hitting your 10k steps a day. That is a minimum you should aim for. If you are able and indeed wish, because it is optional, I would urge you to start some exercise. Anything, you don't have to go mad but anything you do will boost your energy and your metabolism. You will also feel better as those endorphins kick in. This is advice. You will lose weight without exercise, but remember marginal gains! Every little bit helps.

THE FRESHPLAN FRESH FOOD PELOS DIET

I am going into branding overload now. I almost called it the Freshtastic diet, but that was a step too far. In phase 1, I gave you a plan and specific recipes. In phase 2, I give you a template and some simple rules to follow. I have found that everyone is different in what they like to eat and as I firmly believe food is something you have to enjoy, then by giving you control of what you eat, you are far more likely to succeed.

You are going to find this so easy to follow, highly enjoyable and the results will shock you. You will never be hungry and probably, because most people tell me this, won't believe that losing weight can be this easy. On the cover of this book, I call the Freshplan Diet a revolution but in truth, it is more a revelation.

The premise of the Freshplan Fresh Food Diet is that you eat the way nature intended you to eat and your body works the way it is programmed to work. When this happens, your body will normalise and repair itself. A human body that is fed the right fuel and performs to its optimum levels will not get fat and will maintain your health.

Your natural state is one of wellbeing and high energy. This is nothing new. It is sadly something that social evolution has taken away from us. Getting back to the basics of nutrition is a cure for many health and weight issues. Certainly, if everyone followed a fresh food diet, there would be no obesity problem. We get fat because we turn our back on millions of years of evolution and feed our bodies the complete opposite of what it needs to keep us healthy.

What you will do is flip the make-up of your diet from manmade to natural, fresh real food. That does not mean exclusively but the overwhelming majority of the food you eat (90% plus) will be natural food. If you do that, you will get thin and stay thin for life. It is a fact of human biology, psychology, anthropology, sociology, physiology and any other -ology relating to mankind. There is not a doctor, scientist or academic in the world (unless they are on a big food companies' payroll) who can possibly disagree with that statement.

POST DETOX, 2+1

When you have finished the detox, either 7 days or 14 days, you will follow the PELOS 2+1 plan as set out below.

WEEKS 1 to 4

Supplements	Breakfast	Lunch	Dinner	Snacks
MON Probiotic tablet Garlic Tablet	Pelos Green Power Smoothie (1)	Fresh food smoothie	Fresh food dinner Dessert	Piece of Fresh Fruit
TUES Probiotic tablet Garlic Tablet	Pelos Green Power Smoothie (1)	Fresh food smoothie	Fresh food dinner Dessert	Handful of nuts, unsalted or flavoured

WEDS **Prob** **tablet** **Garlic** **Tablet**	Pelos Green Power Smoothie (1)	Fresh food smoothie	Fresh food dinner Fresh food dinner Dessert	Piece of Fresh Fruit
THURS **Prob** **tablet** **Garlic** **Tablet**	Pelos Green Power Smoothie (1)	Fresh food smoothie	Fresh food dinner Dessert	Piece of Fresh Fruit
FRI **Prob** **tablet** **Garlic** **Tablet**	Pelos Green Power Smoothie (1)	Fresh food smoothie	Fresh food dinner Dessert	Handful of Nuts, unsalted or flavoured
SAT **Prob** **tablet** **Garlic** **Tablet**	Pelos Green Power Smoothie (1)	Fresh food smoothie	Fresh food dinner Dessert	SOD IT reward
SUN **Prob** **tablet** **Garlic** **Tablet**	Pelos Green Power Smoothie (1)	Fresh food smoothie	Fresh food dinner Dessert	Piece of Fresh Fruit

<u>**NOTES**</u>	Ensure You drink lots of water, 6 pints minimum a day. Take probiotic first thing and garlic, tasteless and odourless. 1 x coffee with skimmed milked, or 2 x tea skimmed milk daily. NO ALCOHOL PERMITTED (1 glass of wine or beer as sod it Saturday reward). NO FOOD AFTER 7pm

You will have a PELOS POWER SMOOTHIE for breakfast and a fresh fruit smoothie for lunch and you now start eating real food again. That is a key distinction to make. Fresh food is real food and manufactured food (in the main) is fake food because it lacks nutrients. There is a wide range of smoothie recipes on the Freshplan website at www.freshplan.com.

2+1 is a very simple plan but why complicate matters? Easy, losing weight is easy if you stick to this. You will do it, have lots of energy and start to be healthier than ever. The food plan works every time.

You will need to use the Freshplan Mindset to make sure you stick to it but when you do, you your life will turn around. Eating mostly fresh, real food will do the job for you. There is no need for crazy, complicated diets, no need for pills and certainly no need for surgery. The Freshplan Mindset and the Freshplan PELOS Diet is all you need. You can't and won't fail with this is combination. 2+ 1 is really straight forward.

You need to continue with the probiotic tablet and introduce a daily garlic capsule. I am not a big fan of tablets but garlic is so good for you that taking it daily without the smell is a sociable thing to do.

- **Breakfast,** we are sticking with the PELOS POWER SMOOTHIE. This sets you up for the day.
- **Lunch,** you can have a smoothie of your choice from the list or you can make your own, BUT it must contain only fresh fruit and vegetables.
- **Dinner,** you can eat a fresh food dinner and dessert (see below)
- **Dessert,** fresh fruit, natural yoghurts
- **Snack,** there is a designated snack, which you can eat any time before 7pm.

Fresh Food Dinner

This is the key meal of the day. Remember, you must eat before 7pm. You need to eat only fresh food, real food and whole foods. Call it what you like but you need to eat foods that are in their natural state. This is the key to the Freshplan PELOS Diet. Your evening meal should consist of:

- **Protein,** 25% fresh lean meat or fish. This should be unprocessed and not cooked in anything other than extra virgin olive oil. You need to avoid meat with lots of fat. White meat is better, although red meat with the fat trimmed is perfectly fine a couple of times a week.

- **Vegetables or Salads,** 25% pile them on. No dressing on the salads, as many fresh vegetables and salads as you can get. They are great, and you will feel fuller for longer with them.
- **Carbohydrates,** 25% you need carbs in your diet but manage them carefully. Pasta and rice, switch to wholegrain from white. Avoid white bread; avoid all bread if possible. Potatoes, they are perfectly fine as long as they are prepared correctly; no frying, but you can be inventive.

Your plate should always be structured this way:

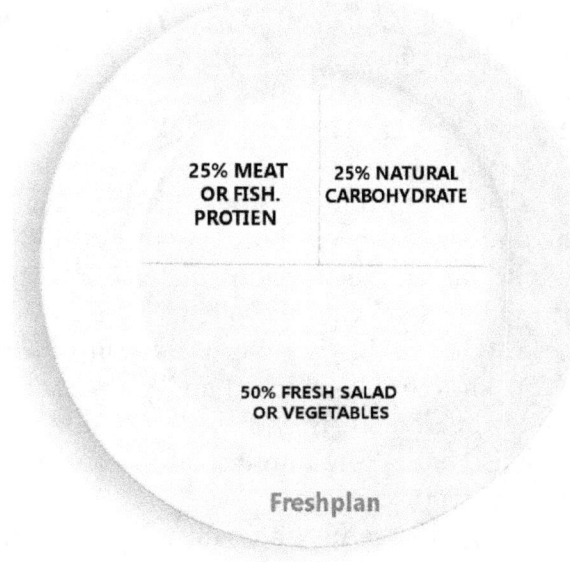

25% MEAT OR FISH. PROTIEN

25% NATURAL CARBOHYDRATE

50% FRESH SALAD OR VEGETABLES

Freshplan

Portion Sizes

If you are hungry and want more, add more vegetables only! This is the only one of the three categories you can have extra. No extras of the other sections. You can eat as much salad and vegetables as you like, as long as it is not prepared with any oils or you don't add any sauces or anything to them. This is very important. You can really enjoy preparing food.

SOME IDEAS FOR PREPARING YOUR EVENING MEAL

If you can cook, then you will love the scope that fresh food offers. If you don't, can't or can't be bothered, then you can make life easy for yourself.

Freshplan Cooking Tip: Buy a Wok

One of the things I do is throw everything in a wok and stir fry everything. Use only extra virgin olive oil. You can get versions that are infused with garlic, chilli and various other natural delights. Chinese style cooking is superb. Use only fresh food and lean protein, like chicken and prawns. You can buy pre-prepared stir-fry mixes, throw it in, add the meat or fish and a few minutes later, you have great tasting fast food.

Be very careful with sauces but you are OK with a teaspoon or two of soy sauce or fish sauce. You can't go wrong and there is a world of flavours waiting for you. Garlic, ginger, spring onion (the holy trinity of Chinese cooking) provide you with so much scope. You can add chilli and just about any vegetables. You can make fried rice but remember the portion size; only 25% of the total should be rice. You genuinely can have a wok meal every day for a week and not have anything the same or even similar. Part of the fun is experimenting. There will be Freshplan PELOS wok recipes on the website, www.Freshplan.com.

Protein, Meat and Fish

You can do so much with meat and fish: grill, oven bake, and pan fry, in extra virgin olive oil. Make sure the meat is lean and try to limit red meat to twice a week. Fish is so good for you and easy to prepare. Fresh fish with spices, wrapped in foil with some lemon and olive oil is simply divine. Make sure you stick to lean meat and prepare it right. Adding hot meat or fish to cold salads is a great tip. Of course, eggs are a great source of protein and you can do a million things with eggs but omelettes are amazing, because you can add so much. If you buy mince, get 5% fat mince. Less fat, the better. Chicken breast, remove the skin, and other meat, like gammon, trim the fat.

Vegetables and salads

There is not much to say. There is such a huge amount of fresh vegetables and salads to choose from. The choice is yours. One thing I will say is that fresh is best. Frozen veg is not as nutritious as fresh and the sooner you eat after peeling or preparation the better. If you can't eat fresh, then frozen is second best. I would not advise you to eat any tinned vegetables. Try to eat them as fresh as possible. Also, be aware of pre-prepared ready-to-eat salads; they have dressing or added sugar. They simply love adding sugar to healthy looking foods!

Carbohydrates, Rice, Pasta and Potatoes

You can eat carbs, moderately, but you need them in your diet, as long as they are balanced and prepared right. Rice and pasta are fine in modest amounts but adopt the white-out principle. By this I mean, do not eat anything white; switch to brown. This means rice and pasta, whole-grain only. Quinoa is a great alternative to rice. Couscous too but avoid flavoured versions. I bet you will hardly notice the difference but nutritionally, white and brown are poles apart.

Potatoes are fine to eat in moderation. The problem comes when you start frying them in vegetable oils but on their own, you can eat potatoes baked, mashed and boiled. As long as you do not exceed the ratio and don't fry them or roast them, they are a good source of fibre and carbohydrate. Don't add butter or anything bad to them and they will do you good. Take away the extra fat and deep frying, and a baked potato is an exceptionally healthy low calorie, high fibre food that offers significant protection against cardiovascular disease and cancer.

Spuds are a very good source of vitamin B6 and a good source of potassium, copper, vitamin C, manganese, phosphorus, niacin, dietary fibre, and pantothenic acid. They get a bad rap because of chips but potatoes are a fresh vegetable. A baked potato with low sugar beans or low fat cottage cheese is a great meal. Try sweet potatoes as an alternative. They are great tasting, and they are full of nutrition.

Where to begin with sweet potatoes? They are your secret weapon. They are full of vitamins, minerals and antioxidants, anti-inflammatory nutrients and blood sugar-regulating nutrients. They are potatoes but with more flavour and they are better for you. Try sweet potato mash, sweet potato wedges or even sweet potato chips; you will love it. See fish and chips below. **Important:** Always prepare fresh, never frozen or oven chips!

Desserts

Why should we forgo dessert? The beauty of this is you don't. You just have to be sensible. Fruit is so nice. Strawberries, all sweet berries, fruit salad, eat what you want. You can have it with zero fat natural yoghurt. You will enjoy it and it is full of nutrition. Tinned prunes is a great desert but this must be in fruit juice. Pitted prunes take the hassle of the stone away. Mix with zero fat yoghurt and you have a great dessert.

One thing that goes against the grain, Muller Light yoghurts. This is processed food but it is very low in calories and it will give you that sweet taste you miss. Only one a day maximum and, ideally, not every day. You may be shocked but we are eating mainly fresh food, mainly not exclusively!

Popular Favourites

You can search the internet for fresh food recipes. There are thousands of them. We feature plenty on the Freshplan.com website. There are literally thousands of options, but as long as you stick to fresh food and avoid adding fats and dressings, you will be fine. Make sure you cut out all added sugar. Sugar is bad, bad, bad. Here are a few popular favourite dishes you may wish to try.

Fish Chips and Peas, Freshplan Style

I promised you fish and chips. Well, here is how you make it without cheating. A filet of fish, cod, haddock or plaice, in fact, any fish will do. Pan fry it and squeeze lemon juice over the fish. Now the clever part, the chips. Peel your potatoes and cut into chips. Part boil them. Drain them and then place on a baking tray, drizzle on olive oil and cook in oven, like you would oven chips. I have a dry fry, which works really well. You will be surprised how, with salt and vinegar, this tastes like chips. Try with sweet potatoes for a different flavour. Add peas, boiled garden peas, and there you go, fish, chips, and peas.

Fancy a Bag of Crisps?

Peel some potatoes and use a mandolin to finely slice. Place them individually on a plate that you can microwave. Drizzle olive oil and put in the microwave. 3 minutes on full, turn over another 1 to

2 minutes, and they will be crispy. Pinch of salt, there you go.

Roast Potatoes / Roast Dinner

Very easy, part boil potatoes and roast with a light drizzle of extra virgin olive oil. Great to serve with chicken and vegetables. For gravy, I use an OXO cube and thicken it with tomato puree and add a splash of Worcestershire sauce.

Cottage Pie

My favourite fresh food meal, because it doesn't feel like diet food but healthy comfort food. Cook onions and mushrooms in a pan, add 5% mince, season, add tinned tomatoes and, possibly, a splash of Worcestershire sauce. Garlic, good for you, adds flavour. Put in a pie dish, put mash on top and cook in the oven. Serve with plenty of fresh vegetables.

Spaghetti Bolognaise

I have this all the time using lean 5% mince. Tomatoes, fresh and tinned, onion mushrooms. Garlic, good for you, adds flavour. Add herbs; coriander is really nice, fresh of course. Serve with wholegrain spaghetti.

Chilli Con Carne

Same base as spag bol, add chilli powder, fresh chillies and kidney beans (if tinned in water) but fresh is better. Serve with brown rice. This is superb!

There are so many things you can do. Make cottage pie, shepherd's pies, you are not limited. In fact, a new world of food and tastes have been opened up for you. There are loads of recipes for you. Yes, you guessed it, more on our website www.freshplan.com.

Exceptions to the rule

Every rule has exceptions. There are some processed foods, though not many, you can eat that are perfectly fine.

- **Baked Beans** (reduced sugar and salt) you may be surprised but baked beans are a great source of protein and they are good for you. Make sure you get the lowest sugar and salt content
- **Tinned Tomatoes / Tomato Puree -** great for sauces and easy.
- **Canned Salmon / Tuna** (in water) - easy and good source of protein
- **Greek yoghurt, 0% fat** really good for you, natural yoghurt, but must be zero fat. Great to have with fruit as a dessert.
- **Tinned Prunes, in fruit juice** - very good for the digestion. Great with zero fat, natural yoghurt. Try to have these once a week, if you like them. Only eat food you like. That is the important thing to remember, always!
- **Muller Light Yoghurt -** this is the item that proves all rules have exceptions. You can

have ONE Muller light as a dessert. Low calories and variable flavour. Limit yourself to one, never two.

- **Low fat cottage cheese -** packed full of protein and nutrients. If you like it, once a week it is fine. Low fat essential.

Sod-it Saturday Rewards

Until you hit your target weight, you must control your rewards. You MUST have a reward but until you hit your target weight, you must be very careful not to go overboard and undo the great work you have done. So be very conscious of what you are having. For example, you may have a bag of crisps, a small chocolate bar or a glass of wine. But have one of those, not all. Plan your rewards and look forward to them. When you get to your target weight, you will be able to broaden the scope of rewards, but the trick is to get to your weight, rather than taking backward steps to slow you down.

Snacks

The plan includes snacks, which are optional. You do not need to have them, only if you have a strong craving. No harm will be done by a few almonds or a piece of fruit but you should try to remain on the plan. We all have 'snack attacks'; this is normal.

You Will Achieve Your Objectives With 2+1

2+1 is the quickest way to get to your target weight. You will not be hungry. True hunger is listening to your stomach, not the cravings in your head. You will have cravings but not true hunger. Keep journaling and the habits; make sure you weigh yourself, same time, and with as few clothes as possible.

You will have setbacks, but do not give up. This plan will get you to your target weight and it will also give you plenty of energy. Your nutrition will be so improved, you should see many benefits, better skin, better hair and a brighter more positive mood.

STICK TO THE PLAN. Do not give up. You are eating food your body was designed to eat. This is the most important change you need to make in your life to become the correct weight and maintain it. We have, generally, lost the ability to listen to our bodies.

Recognise hunger, embrace it. Hunger from the stomach. This is the relationship you need to have with food, food for fuel, not as the subject of an addiction. You must learn to eat to live, not live to eat. When you become the former, you will see how the latter has been the cause of your weight, health and energy issues for too long.

I cannot stress enough that the key is to listen to your body. Eating only when you are hungry, eating just enough, not overeating and eating what is nutritionally required by your body is the secret to weight, energy and good health.

It actually isn't a secret but it seems to have been forgotten, as the size of the average human waistline will testify. Manage your food, don't let it manage you. That is, my friends, as simple as it needs to be. When you realise that and make that second nature, it is plain sailing. You now know everything I do, and losing weight will be as easy for you.

You have no excuses; losing weight is easy now. You know why you have failed in the past. Your Mindset wasn't right. Now, you have the mind management tools in place to go for it with a positive Mindset and complete control of the outcome. If you want to do it, and clearly you do, you will do it.

This plan will reduce your weight and fuel you with bags of energy. As I said in Chapter 1, it is your Mindset that will determine whether or not to succeed. But you have all the tools to achieve your objectives. You have the Objectives defined, the Strategy in place, and a whole range of Tactics to employ.

Eat only when you are hungry and ensure that you apply the WWW (What, When and Why) test to the food that passes your lips. Deal with cravings with the POWER technique and use the energy that the PELOS plan gives you to keep your motivation high. Your journal is vital. Do not ever let it slide. Keep with it, make it a habit and it will serve you well.

Results will become visible to others and you will become a minor celebrity within your social, work and living circles. People will want to talk about your weight loss and will want some of the feel-good magic. When you feel down or demotivated, look beyond it and keep your eyes on the prize. They are simply obstacles on the path to happiness. The Freshplan works. It gets you thin but it also makes you healthy and gives you more energy than you have had for a long time and, as we know, energy powers success.

You are on the journey from failure to success, from fat to thin, and from despair to happiness. Getting there though is just the start.

Chapter 19
Freshplan lifelong weight management

When you go on a diet and reach your target weight, what next? Far too many people think they have done the job and go back to their old ways. But it is not a circle. As we know, circles are vicious, so you need to switch to weight management, rather than a weight loss strategy. Once you have got to your target weight, keeping it off is easier still, of course, with the right Mindset.

When you started reading, I spoke about the new improved version of you. You should be the same person but with upgraded mindware, one programmed to eat to live, able to effectively manage the hungry goblin and someone who is able to control their weight. I would be delighted to hear from you. If you have achieved great results, drop me an email, carl@freshplan.com.

You will have much more energy, which powers a positive outlook on life. In a nutshell, you will look and feel great. This, though, is not your final destination. A great saying is:

"Happiness is not a destination, it is a journey of a lifetime."

That is true because now that you have achieved your target weight and fulfilled your weight loss goals, you are not going to turn around and go back to where you started. You are not that person anymore. You packed up and left 'Fatsville' and moved to 'Happytown', which is your forever home.

"Never go back!"

Let's be blunt. Why would you ever want to go back? I am probably stating the obvious but for the vast majority of people, the idea of going back to their old life is horrifying! But you will need to do more than just hope. You need to make sure that happens.

I said that no one can truly be happy being fat and even if you thought you were a happy fatty, I'm willing to wager you are happier now that you have reached your ideal weight. Looking in the mirror and feeling good is a feeling I, for one, had not had the benefit of for many years. What you have done in losing weight is fantastic and the feeling of wellbeing and high energy is your reward. Your goal in life is to make sure that this is the person you will always be; the new you is here to stay. You are no longer on a diet. You have, however, made a lifestyle change and you are someone who is in control of their weight.

It stands to reason that if you stop all your good habits, stop watching What, When and Why you eat, you will get fat again. Another age old adage is:

"Prevention is easier than cure."

Of course, it is far easier to not get fat than to get fat and have to lose it all again. If you allow yourself to get fat again, then you will be that lacklustre, demotivated, miserable person and having enjoyed the good life, you will be really down about letting your goblin brain take over again and run your life. That said, if you have done it once, you can do it again but there is no need to ride the big yoyo rollercoaster. Life is plain sailing from here. Managing weight, armed with the Freshplan Mindset and Freshplan PELOS Diet, is now second nature to you.

Everything you have followed to get you to your target weight will keep you there. The first thing to do is to revise your goals and objectives. Your goals may be simply to stay within at your ideal weight, but you may want to introduce new goals to maintain your energy, motivation, or even to get physically fit through exercise.

Having gotten your weight under control, you may wish to set goals in other parts of your life. You have a limitless supply of energy, if you continue to eat well, which will power you towards success. Personal Energy Level Output is the key to Success in all aspects of your life, a goal you should strive for, for life.

Your objective is to stay within your threshold weight, both upper and lower. Being too thin is just as bad as being too fat. You, therefore, need to determine your upper and lower weight parameters. If you become underweight, well, you don't need my help to address that particular issue. If you breakthrough your upper limit, then you need to lose some weight, using the tools you have at your disposal. That is a reactive strategy, and of course, it is better to be proactive.

PROACTIVE WEIGHT MANAGEMENT STRATEGIES

There is no hard and fast rules about the ideal strategy for weight management, because everyone is different, both physically and mentally. What works for one person may not for another. For me, I find it easier to have zero of anything, rather than one, which leads to two and three. Not starting is easier than stopping. Find what works for you.

DO NOT UNDO ALL THE GOOD WORK YOU HAVE DONE!

This is important. Just because you are thin, your physiology hasn't changed. You will get fat much quicker than it took you to get thin! The first thing you should do is replace your lunch smoothie with a meal. I would advise very strongly that you continue to have a PELOS smoothie for breakfast because of the nutritional and energy benefits. It will also fill you up and release protein slowly, making you feel fuller for longer.

For lunch, you should have something light. Stick with fresh food. If you continue to eat mostly fresh real food, you will find keeping your weight down easy! Of course, you can relax a bit and live it up, but control and moderation is the key. There are some other golden rules that will help make keeping your weight loss easy:

- **Eat fresh real food** as much as possible and regard all manufactured food as bad, fattening, and off limits.
- **Weigh yourself** religiously EVERY MORNING. Even if you don't want to see bad news, make it a habit.
- **Drink water** first thing in a morning and throughout the day.
- **Only eat when you are hungry**, do not eat when you are full, and live by the HARA HACHI BU principle. *"Eight parts of a full stomach sustain the man; the other two sustain the doctor."*
- **Control the liquid calories**. You will consume far more than you realise if you do not consciously monitor them. Alcohol is a big potential pitfall. You will need to decide what you do, but the less you consume, the better your life, weight and your health will be. That is a fact but you have free will and the choice is yours.
- **Keep moving!** Exercise of any kind will help. As a minimum, you should aim for 10k steps a day.
- **Never say sod-it again!** You can very easily become complacent. One of the main reasons people slip back is because they become complacent. They celebrate losing weight and never stop celebrating then they live a sod-it existence with the old excuses, and the goblin takes over. Don't allow that to happen.

- **Remember you are in control**. Personal responsibility and self-discipline will determine lifelong success.
- **Keep writing in your journal**, it really helps. This is will keep your Mindset positive and your motivation high.
- **Energise your life,** make your main focus in life keeping your personal energy levels high, which powers success.

All the techniques discussed in section 1 will help. Keep practising them. Read more books, never stop learning. Let me share with you what I call the **Arkwright Review.**

I used to watch the BBC TV comedy programme Open All Hours as a kid, with Ronnie Barker as a money grabbing, stuttering shopkeeper, obsessed with Nurse Gladys Emmanuelle. The character was called Arkwright who, at the end of every show, would stand outside his shop and review the day. No more than a few minutes but what a great concept this is. The last thing I do before I go to bed, I spend a few minutes at the end of the day to look back at the day; what I did well, what I did bad and what I will do better tomorrow. I don't always write this down but it is a powerful tool which will keep your mind in focus. Give it a go. Small changes, big differences.

In terms of your eating plan to manage weight, you will find what works for you, but here are a few ideas:

THE FRESHPLAN 5:2 PLAN

This is one of the most popular plans that works for people. For five days, you eat fresh food with a PELOS breakfast smoothie, rigidly observing the fresh food only rules. For two days, you eat what you want. People who work Monday to Friday find this works particularly well for them. Of course, you need to keep an eye on the scales to see if it works for you.

THE FRESHPLAN + SOD-IT SATURDAY (6:1)

This works best for me. I like the discipline, the build-up to Saturday and to get back on it. This is where I follow the Freshplan for six days. A breakfast smoothie, healthy fresh food for lunch and dinner with fruit, nuts and seeds and snacks. Limit coffee and have no more than one with caffeine with skimmed milk. Drink plenty of water. Stay disciplined but on Saturday I have a big sod-it Saturday reward (it can be any day you choose). There is not much damage you can do in one day if you stick to the plan rigidly for 6 days.

1 WEEK A MONTH

I know a few people who swear by this, but I don't particularly like it. They eat what they like and they detox for a week every month. It manages the waistline but I prefer to keep the nutrients giving me energy. As I said, everyone is different and looks at life differently. This may work for you. Certainly, if you go away and comeback a bit heavy, you can detox on smoothies until your weight normalises again.

MOSTLY FRESH FOOD

You may adopt the fresh food plan as your plan for life and only sod-it on special occasions, like social events, celebrations or holidays. Make it a way of life. For some people, this is a step too far and for others it is easy. Certainly, if you agree that it is not just about weight but nutrition and energy, this will serve you well. Someone said to me that in trying to live longer, you can be in danger of not living at all. I know what he means. Life is for living and to be enjoyed. You need to strike a balance.

Find what works for you and suits your lifestyle. But you have the knowledge, the power, and the tools to successfully manage your weight.

SHARE THE MAGIC, MAKE PEOPLE HAPPY!

You are a success and people will be inspired by you. If you can do it, they will want to do it. They will admire you and see you as a success. The new you will be inspirational and it may seem an odd thing to say but you will take on celebrity-like status in the circles you interact. People will want to know how you did it and you can go one step further by taking on the role of mentor.

A great way of keeping you in the right Mindset is to become a Freshplan Mentor. This is where you help people lose weight by giving both guidance and support. You can do this on an informal basis or make money as a Freshplan Accredited Mentor. Details can be found on the website www.freshplan.com.

The Freshplan Diet by Carl Harris

Chapter 20
This is the first day of the rest of your life

That is it, the end, but it is really only the beginning. Thank you for reading and I hope you have enjoyed it and, above all, have lost weight and changed your outlook on life. I would love to hear from you. My email is carl@freshplan.com and there will be lots more on our website www.freshplan.com.

This is the first day of the rest of your life. A life lived thin, healthy and with an abundance of energy. No-one knows how long we have left but we have a fair idea. I want to enjoy every day and make sure I have as many of them as I can, of course, we all do. Being happy is by far the best way to live life. Energy is the key to a happy and healthy life.

Having been addicted to sugar, Diet Coke and a sedentary existence, there is no way I am ever going to be fat again. With the Freshplan, you can create an upgraded version of you that will ensure your life is just better. The Mindset, the habits and motivation, all powered by your personal energy levels, will have beneficial knock-on effects in other areas of your life.

Similarly, if you allow yourself to slip back to your old ways, you will find the same effect in reverse with negativity cascading into other aspects of your world. The power to dictate the direction your life takes is in your hands. You really have the power.

I have not mentioned it for a while but 85% of people who try to lose weight, fail. So what you have done is a great achievement. You should be very proud but do not look at it as job done. In fact, it is just the start.

When a sportsman becomes World Champion, they do not ease off on the practice and training. They work harder. That feeling of triumph and invincibility is as dangerous as it is powerful. If you become lazy or complacent, you can very quickly undo the good work you have done.

Losing weight is an uphill climb. You have to put effort into every step. Putting it back on is the opposite. It is downhill and you can freewheel backwards with no effort at all, very easily, without even trying. You must make sure you keep pushing and looking at it in this way shows that just standing still (maintaining your weight) also requires effort. If you let the brake off, you quickly roll downhill.

That is why you must never let your Mindset revert back to your old one. Everything the Freshplan has taught you are skills for life. Use them every day. That doesn't mean you are on a diet for the rest of your life but it does mean you have to keep monitoring your weight and taking action to make sure you never ever go back to the person you used to be.

I said it at the start. Look at the Freshplan as an investment in the people you love and who love you and never lose sight of that. Do it for you but, above all, do it for them. It will not be easy but always remember this: life is better when you live it the hard way, and winners never quit because quitters never win.

Thank you.

Carl Harris